BUT I CAN'T EAT THAT

By

Heidi Passow

Kitchen-Tested Recipes for People with Multiple Allergies

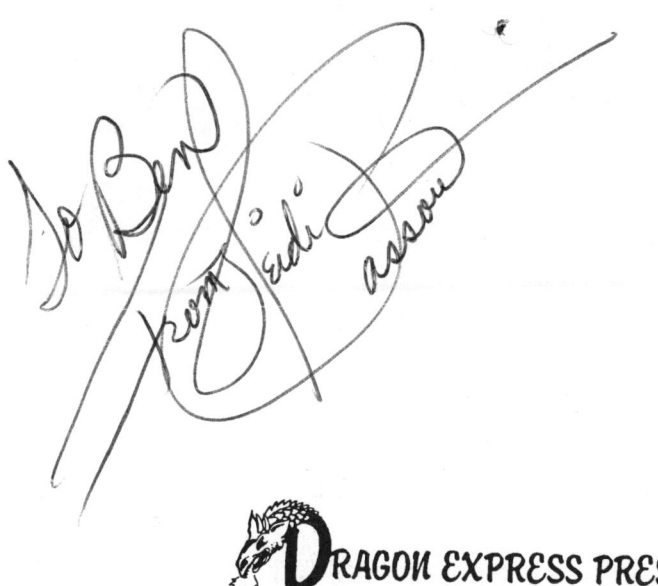

DRAGON EXPRESS PRESS

Copyright 1994 by Heidi Passow
Cover Art Work and Design By: Dan Irwin
Logo and Wheaten Design By: Heidi Passow
Logo and Wheaten Art Work By: Peter C. Lutjen

All rights reserved. No part of this Cookbook can be reproduced in any form by electronic, mechanical, photocopy, recording, information storage or retrieval system, without written permission from the publisher, except by a reviewer who wishes to quote brief passages in a review. This Cookbook is not intended as a substitute for proper diagnoses and treatment. Because each person is unique, we urge you to already know your own medical status before using this cookbook. The author and the publisher are not responsible for adverse affects or consequences resulting from the use of any preparations, processes or suggestions in this book. Any slights of people or organizations are unintentional.

Published By:
DRAGON EXPRESS PRESS
2604 Saybrook Rd.
Cleveland, Ohio
44118-4722

Publisher's Cataloging in Publication
(Prepared by Quality Books Inc.)

Passow, Heidi.
   But I can't eat that : kitchen tested recipes for people with multiple allergies / by Heidi Passow.
   p. cm.
   Includes index.
   Preassigned LCCN: 93-090578.
   ISBN 0-963-7260-9-9

   1. Food allergy--Diet therapy--Recipes.   I. Title.

RC588.D53P37 1993   641.563'1
                                              QB193-992

1 2 3 4 5 6 7 8 9 10

"Printed and bound in the United States of America"

DEDICATED TO JONATHAN
By eating the foods recommended by the Dragon Express
you will live long and prosper.

BUT I CAN'T EAT THAT

TABLE OF CONTENTS

	Page
INTRODUCTION	1-2
CHAPTER 1 OFFERING HELPFUL IDEAS HOW TO USE THIS COOKBOOK IMPORTANCE OF FRESH FOODS ASPECTS OF MENU PLANNING TRAVEL INGREDIENTS AND SUBSTITUTIONS	3-21
CHAPTER 2 PROTEINS	22-80
CHAPTER 3 CARBOHYDRATES	81-109
CHAPTER 4 FRUITS AND VEGETABLES	110-130
CHAPTER 5 SOUPS SAUCES SEASONINGS	131-156
CHAPTER 6 SWEET MEAL TOPPERS	157-176
CHAPTER 7 COMPANY'S COMING (Recipes for people with no allergies)	177-194
Appendices	195-221
Safe and Accessible Foods	195-197
Agencies and People to Contact	198-199
Recommended Reading	200-201
References	202-203
Addendum on Illness (Recipes benefiting people with these medical problems)	207-211
Index	212-223

PREFACE

WHY I WROTE THIS BOOK

Ever since I can remember (that is age 7) I've suffered from headaches, nausea and migraines. No one could diagnose any problem, but I was assured as I became older I would grow out of them. Instead, symptoms grew out of control. After becoming totally frustrated, I was sent to "THE ALLERGIST." At first I was so upset to find I was allergic AND sensitive to so many items that I didn't believe him. Finally I decided that I had nothing to loose and tried eliminating food items one at a time. The result was astounding. Now after 11 years of having my allergies and sensitivity under control, I am completely headache free (except when I cheat). My son started from day one with allergies, (though different ones than myself) but by then I was educated about controlling them. Knowing how to identify and handle his reactions has helped with this problem. FACT: Every 7-10 years one does grow in or out of allergies.

People tend to learn to control their allergies by eating the same thing for breakfast, lunch and dinner. I did this and did indeed feel 100% better. But, it was very boring. Adding tolerated spices and colorful foods, I created <u>But I Can't Eat That</u>. Meals became fun and easier to eat in the prescribed manner. I could even entertain again! I do carry "safe" foods with me wherever I go. No one has objected to bringing my own food once I explain my predicament. People comment "Oh, that really smells delicious. What is it?" OR "That looks very tasty." I comment, I am visiting to enjoy the pleasure of their <u>company</u> (not their food) and it was the truth!

■ Gourmet

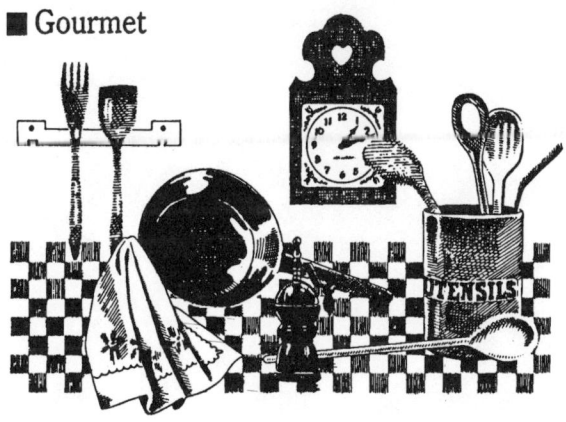

ACKNOWLEDGEMENTS

My Loving Thanks to Richard, my husband and Jonathan, my son for whom I wrote this book, and Jean, my mother for the help and support on this project. My Thanks to all the people who helped and encouraged me. Some with just their words and others with their patience and expertise. Special thanks to Jean Cunnings, MA, Pauline Degenfelder, Ph.D., Gary A. Katz, Marianne Calabrese Kukec, Peter Lutjen, John Miller, Ph.D., Office Staff at Dr. H. Schwartz, M.D., Allergist, Estelle M. Parker, Mary Alice Passow, Tom Satyshur Jr. and Pearl Urban.

BUT I CAN'T EAT THAT

INTRODUCTION

I Will AND CAN DO IT

Today people consume prepared, frozen, overly flavored, colored and preserved food products, without realizing that these ingredient(s) may be making them ill. Some 15-20% of the United States population has allergy reactions (my son and myself included). Even the simplest foods can cause adverse effects. This cookbook can help you ease your way out of allergy reactions and targets 14 most commonly combined (ingredients) allergy problems. Review Addendum on Illness for more suggestions. Recipes in <u>But I Can't Eat That</u> have none of these allergy ingredients and also avoid commercial food products. The recipes are easy to prepare, involve little time and are self adjusting for a customized cooking mode. I've also listed allergy and chemical free products to help cut down on your time spent cooking. (See Safe and Accessible Foods.) Utilize them in your own personal way to control what you eat and there by control the allergy reactions that definitely leave you "hung-over."

This cookbook has healthful food suggestions for people with multiple allergies. The point of this book is to become symptom or reaction free. Some allergies are lifelong with no cure. Others are just enough to disrupt normal life. Both need to be addressed and taken care of to enjoy an improved life style.

As a person whose diet is restricted, I discovered it takes a great deal of courage to start and maintain dietary changes. <u>But I Can't Eat That</u> will push you towards a livable goal. If you benefit from just one idea in this book, it will have made it worth my effort!

For people with allergies, foods need to be created from scratch as much as possible. Fresh foods are a must if food preservatives are to be eliminated. Food for people with mold allergies need to be cooked and eaten within a 18 to 24 hour period. No dried foods are allowed, since they contain preservatives and carry mold spores. Only you know what your limits and requirements are. This type of cooking demands time, patience and a drive to feel better. You must learn what health problems are real for you. Build up your immune system by staying clear of the allergens. If chocolate contributes to your allergy reactions, eliminate it. Treat it as a poison, for it truly will make you ill.

<u>Let your doctor</u> put together a list of requirements for your specific problems. Many of the recipes in this cookbook will meet the requirements. Check the foods on the Vitamin List to strengthen your immune system properly, along with your regular vitamins pills.

BUT I CAN'T EAT THAT

I WILL AND CAN DO IT (Cont.)
Test your limitations every six months to keep your chart updated. Less severe cases might want to test more often. You know you are on the right track when you can tolerate a wee bit more than you could the last time. Then you are headed in the right direction and your eating regime is working!!! (Yes, it is slow. But, you must take slow improvement as encouragement!)

1. Know what ingredients are on your hit list!
   It is important to READ ALL LABELS.

2. You must determine to what extent you are sensitive. Only you can determine this. For example, if you cannot tolerate dried teas because of mold, you may or may not tolerate dried spices. This is important to your cooking tastes, so testing your sensitivity to spices should be your number one priority.

3. If you haven't read it on the label OR haven't made it your self OR have not gotten the assurance from the chef of the establishment, don't eat it. Better to be SAFE than SICK.

Many basic cooking ingredients <u>can</u> be made from scratch. Make ahead meals are easy if you have a freezer and some extra time. The advantage to this is knowing what ingredients are in these meals. You can eat them without dissecting the ingredients first. Put aside one day (or a block of time) to do preparing, packaging and freezing foods that agree with you. The health benefits of keeping your blood stream clear (not to mention time saved for the rest of the week!) outweighs the cost of the containers and freezer space.

There are many books on the market covering individual allergies, assuming you only have a "few" allergic foods to avoid (but try finding books that handle <u>multiple allergies</u>). By the time you eliminate the allergic ingredients in these recipes, the result is nothing left to eat. People may have several different allergy problems at the same time for combined eating problems. This means you are only allergic to, say eggs, but milk gives you intestinal problems. I hope this book will help you cope, while giving you ideas on how to devise your own menu game plan. I wish someone had written <u>this</u> cookbook when our family's medical/allergy troubles erupted.

I wish you luck.

Heidi Passow.

Chapter 1

Offering Helpful Ideas

How to use this Cookbook

Importance of Fresh Foods

Aspects of Menu Planning

Vitamins and Minerals

Freezer Storage Times

Peak Seasons for Fresh Foods

Recipe Charts

Non-critic Mayo Spread

Travel

CHAPTER 1
HOW TO USE THIS COOKBOOK

THE IMPORTANCE OF FRESH FOODS

Cook with top quality foods for good taste and color and you will not go wrong. (Even if you do not feel well now.) Fresh foods will produce optimum nutritional value. Using all natural, fresh, wholesome ingredients which you like provides wonderful flavor making it easier to keep on the prescribed regime. This improves your chances of recovering faster. Use the supplied Vitamins and Minerals Chart for an additional boost of what is missing in your particular diet, ie: if you are allergic to dairy you will need a calcium source to pull from. The Chart will tell you what foods carry calcium for consumption in the diet.

To do this locate the freshest butcher, grocery, produce and health food stores in your area. Butcher shops take a while to locate. They must be consistent with their meat products. Consistency. Fresh, Fresh, Fresh. Word of mouth is the best way to locate a better butcher or grocer. Check the Freezer Storage Times Chart for length of holding freezer times after purchasing, packaging and freezing at home.

Open air produce markets are wonderful, but your selection will be limited to seasonal time frames. Today, grocery stores all over the country can get most vegetables and fruits all year round. Use the Peak Seasons for Fresh Foods Chart to do your planning. When in season pick your own fruits and vegetables. This is much fun and very satisfying. The best taste is what you are after. Superb dining!

Don't overlook health food and specialty stores. Entering a health food store for the first time can be overwhelming. You can get a mainstay of products here. Go in with questions in hand. Know what to look for. Have ideas the employees can expand on. A good store will have very knowledgeable people there or will look answers up if they do not know. They should be able to explain differences in products. Are the foods and items well organized and grouped together? Are products easy to find? Is the price and selection good? Do they have an allergy section? If the owner or employee will break down or split packages for testing products, you know you have found the right place to do your shopping. Are they willing to order products for you or find out how you can purchase them? These are all things to consider when looking for helpful specialty stores.

CHAPTER 1

THE IMPORTANCE OF FRESH FOODS (cont.)

David Vitantonio, owner of "Vitality Health Foods" in Willoughby Hills, Ohio says "The quality of the ingredients in health food products is much better today. Health food companies are ready to improve their products quicker than regular companies. They change as soon as they know of a better ingredient. For example, they found out how bad hydrogenated oils were for the body and took them out immediately, adding better oils. Regular companies (not health food companies) have not changed their ingredients for years and years."

ASPECTS OF MENU PLANNING

The recipes in this cookbook are free of chemicals (such as MSG and sulfates), no preservatives, artificial flavorings, coloring or cane sugar. Utilize the Recipe Charts in planing your meals as allergies allow. Locate any recipes that contain the least number of your particular allergens OR use the Ingredients and Substitutions list to convert a part of the recipe to fit your needs by eliminating the allergen and switching it to an item compatible to your system.

Recipes in But I Can't Eat That! have subheadings labeled IDEAS:. These are "safe" ingredients you can add to customize the recipe to your own tastes. The subheading IF: are clauses at the end of the recipes contain items not "safe" or not tolerated by people with allergies. These add-in's may be used for company or other members of the family. This section is to try and ease the workload of making multiple dishes at meal time. Pull your portion out before adding IF items to serve to the rest of the family.

NOTE: Recipes not conducive to prescribed diet should not be used.
Reminder: If you keep chemically and additive free and avoid your allergens for a good period of time, symptoms can and do recede!!

*Here is a sample menu plan developed from
But I Can't Eat That:*

Breakfast
Rice Muffin
Homemade Peanut Butter

Lunch
Steamed Fish
Steamed Vegetables
Steamed Rice

Dinner
*Pounded Chicken Breasts/
steamed or sautéd
Microwaved Zucchini
Brown Rice/Safflower oil and
Sea Salt*

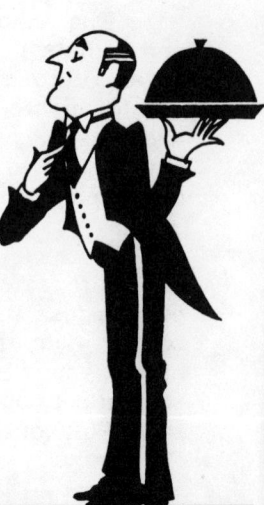

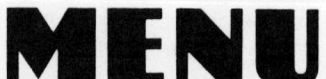

CHAPTER 1

<u>VITAMINS AND MINERALS</u>

Vitamin A	butter, cantaloupe, carrots, dark green and yellow vegetables, parsley, spinach, tomatoes, red pepper
Vitamin B1	fish, lean meat, liver, pork, poultry
Vitamin B2	dark leafy vegetables, lean meat, liver, milk
Vitamin B6	bananas, chicken, peanuts and peanut butter, pork, potatoes, swordfish, tuna, turkey
Vitamin B12	cheese, eggs, fish, liver, meat, milk, seafood
Vitamin C	broccoli, Brussels sprouts, cantaloupe, cauliflower, grapefruit, green and red peppers, natural apple juice, oranges, peas, potatoes, strawberries, tomatoes
Vitamin D	eggs, milk, sunlight
Vitamin E	leafy vegetables, nuts, Safflower Oil, vegetable oil
Vitamin K	cauliflower, leafy vegetables, tomatoes
Calcium	almonds, butter, cheese, citrus fruits, dark leafy vegetables, dried beans, milk, salmon with bones, shellfish
Iron	beef, chicken, dark green vegetables, dark molasses, lean meats, liver, oysters, potatoes with skin, shrimp, spinach, turkey
Potassium	(women require more), bananas, butter, fruits, meats, milk, peanuts, pork, raisins, swordfish, turkey, vegetables
Magnesium	green leafy vegetables, meat, milk, nuts

CHAPTER 1

FREEZER STORAGE TIMES
(for 0 degrees Fahrenheit)

1-2 Months	3-4 Months	5-7 Months	8-12 Months
bread	chops	butter	chicken
cake	cookies	duck	juices
fish	homemade pasta	fruit	
ground meat	prepared	nuts	
ice cream	dinners	roasts	
pies	steak	turkey	
soup		vegetables	
stock			

PEAK SEASONS FOR FRESH FOODS
(Best purchase prices. Basic time frame for the U.S.A.)

All year	bananas, beans, broccoli, cabbage, carrots cauliflower, celery, corn, cucumber, grapefruit, grapes, lettuce, onion, oranges, peppers, pineapple, potatoes, radishes, spinach, squash, strawberries, sweet potatoes, tomatoes
January, Feb, March	apples, Brussels Sprouts, pears
April	Brussels Sprouts, eggs and turkey
May	cantaloupe, corn, peaches, plums, strawberries, tomatoes
June, July, August	blackberries, blueberries, cantaloupe, sweet cherries, corn, fresh fish, melons, peaches, pears, plums, tomatoes, watermelon
September	blackberries, cauliflower, corn, grapes, peaches, pears, plums, tomatoes
October November	apples, Brussels sprouts, cantaloupe, cranberries, pears, pumpkin, sweet potatoes, turkey, watermelon, winter squash
December	apples, cranberries, pears, turkey

BUT I CAN'T EAT THAT

RECIPE CHART
X means that ingredient is contained in the recipe.

A=CHEMICALS	F=EGG	K=CORN
B=ARTIFICIAL COLOR	G=YEAST	L=CHICKEN
C=CANE SUGAR	H=BEEF	M=TOMATOES
D=WHEAT	I=MALT OR BARLEY	N=POTATO
E=MILK	J=OATS	

```
                                  A B C D E F G H I J K L M N
BEEF
Beef Chow Mein                   .............X............
Extra Savory Meat Loaf           .............X............
Porcupine Balls                  .............X............
Heidi's Allergy Pot Roast        .............X............
Swiss Steak                      .............X............
Beef Stew                        .............X............
S.O.M. More (Save Our Mouth)     .............X............
Leftover Beef Pie                ......X......X............
Flank Steak                      .............X............
Hamburger                        .............X............
Hamburger Skillet Toss           .............X............
Hamburger Bake                   .............X............
Quick Beef Meal Ideas            ........X....X............
Meat Stuffed Zucchini            .............X.........X..
Pureed Meat                      .............X............
All Homemade Lasagna             ......X.X.X..X.........X..
Allergy Lasagna                  .............X.........X..
CHICKEN
Plain Baked Chicken              .......................X....
Plain Oven Fried Chicken         .......................X....
Plain Microwaved Chicken         .......................X....
Crock Pot Chicken                .......................X....
Marinated Chicken Breasts        .......................X....
No Fuss Chicken Dinner           .......................X....
Quick Chicken                    .......................X....
Hot Chicken Salad                .......................X....
One Step Chicken and Rice        .......................X....
Chicken Pot Pie                  ......X................X....
Breaded Chicken Strips           ......X...X............X....
Chicken and Tomato Casserole     ..........X............X.X..
Allergy Chicken Chow Mein        .......................X....
Chicken and Rice Scrapple        .......................X....
Chicken Fritters                 ...............X............
Rolled Chicken Bundles           .......................X....
Chicken Loaf                     .......................X....
Chicken Rolls                    .......................X....
Chicken Burgers                  .......................X....
Chicken Protein Spread           .......................X....
Chicken Liver Pate               .......................X....
Crispy Chicken Chips             .......................X....
```

RECIPE CHART

X means that ingredient is contained in the recipe.

A=CHEMICALS	F=EGG	K=CORN
B=ARTIFICIAL COLOR	G=YEAST	L=CHICKEN
C=CANE SUGAR	H=BEEF	M=TOMATOES
D=WHEAT	I=MALT OR BARLEY	N=POTATO
E=MILK	J=OATS	

```
                                A B C D E F G H I J K L M N
EGGS
Dunkin Eggs                     . . . . . . . . . X . . . . .
German Pancakes                 . . . . . . X . . X . . . . .
German Apple Pancakes           . . . . . . X . . X . . . . .
Skillet Breakfast               . . . . . . . . . X . . . . X
Jonathan's Allergy Rollups      . . . . . . X . . X . . . . .
FISH
No Turn Basic Fish Formulas     . . . . . . . . . . . . . . .
Baked                           . . . . . . . . . . . . . . .
Baked and Stuffed               . . . . . . . . . . . . . . .
Steamed                         . . . . . . . . . . . . . . .
Steaks                          . . . . . . . . . . . . . . .
Pan Fried                       . . . . . . . . . . . . . . .
Sauce                           . . . . . . . . . . . . . . .
Seafood Pilaf                   . . . . . . . . . . . . . . .
Fish and Spinach Wraps          . . . . . . . . . . . . . . .
Tuna Patties                    . . . . . . . . . . . . . . .
LAMB
Lamb Roast                      . . . . . . . . . . . . . . .
Lamb Chops                      . . . . . . . . . . . . . . .
Lamb Pot Pie                    . . . . . . X . . . . . . . .
Lamb Stew                       . . . . . . . . . . . . . . .
Lamb Wrap                       . . . . . . X . . X . . . . .
Allergy Lamb Loaf               . . . . . . . . . . . . . . .
Lamb Meatballs in White Sauce   . . . . . . . . . . . . . . .
PORK
Basic Pork Chops                . . . . . . . . . . . . . . .
Grilled                         . . . . . . . . . . . . . . .
Pork Tenderloin                 . . . . . . . . . . . . . . .
Roast                           . . . . . . . . . . . . . . .
Just Ribs (Western Spare Ribs)  . . . . . . . . . . . . . . .
Sweet Pork Cutlets              . . . . . . . . . . . . . . .
Allergy Sausage Patties         . . . . . . . . . . . . . . .
Pork Pot Pie with Vegetables    . . . . . . X . . . . . . . .
Pork City Chicken               . . . . . . . . . . . . . . .
Pork Chop Skillet Dinner        . . . . . . . . . . . . . . .
```

BUT I CAN'T EAT THAT

RECIPE CHART
X means that ingredient is contained in the recipe.

A=CHEMICALS	F=EGG	K=CORN
B=ARTIFICIAL COLOR	G=YEAST	L=CHICKEN
C=CANE SUGAR	H=BEEF	M=TOMATOES
D=WHEAT	I=MALT OR BARLEY	N=POTATO
E=MILK	J=OATS	

```
                                    A B C D E F G H I J K L M N
```

VEAL
	A	B	C	D	E	F	G	H	I	J	K	L	M	N
Veal Patties	.	.	.	.	.	.	.	.	.	.	.	.	.	.
Veal Scallopini Caccitore	.	.	.	.	.	.	.	.	.	.	.	X	.	.

TURKEY
	A	B	C	D	E	F	G	H	I	J	K	L	M	N
Turkey Hash	.	.	.	.	.	.	.	.	.	.	X	.	.	X
Ground Turkey	.	.	.	.	.	.	.	.	.	.	.	.	.	.
C/T Meatballs	.	.	.	.	.	.	.	.	.	.	.	.	.	.

MISCELLANEOUS
	A	B	C	D	E	F	G	H	I	J	K	L	M	N
Meat Turnovers	.	.	.	.	.	X	.	.	X	X	.	.	.	.
Heidi's No Cheese Ravioli	.	.	.	.	.	X	.	.	X	.	.	X	.	.

BREADS
	A	B	C	D	E	F	G	H	I	J	K	L	M	N
Basic:French	.	.	.	.	.	X	.	.	.	.	X	.	.	.
Cut Biscuits	.	.	.	.	.	X	.	.	.	.	X	.	.	.
Italian Bread	.	.	.	.	X	.	X	.	.	.	X	.	.	.
Bread Sticks	.	.	.	.	X	.	X	.	.	.	X	.	.	.
Red Bread	.	.	.	.	X	.	X	.	.	.	X	.	.	.
Green Bread	.	.	.	.	X	.	X	.	.	.	X	.	.	.
Orange Bread	.	.	.	.	X	.	X	.	.	.	X	.	.	.
Heavier English Muffin Bread	.	.	.	.	X	X	X	.	.	.	X	.	.	.
Zucchini Bread-brown rice flour	.	.	.	.	.	.	.	X	.	.	.	.	.	.
Zucchini Bread	.	.	.	.	X	X	.	.	.	.	X	.	.	.
Drop Bread	.	.	.	.	X	X	.	.	.	.	X	.	.	.
Rye Tortillas	.	.	.	.	.	.	.	.	.	.	.	.	.	.
Rye Allergy Loaf	.	.	.	.	.	.	.	.	.	.	.	.	.	.
Drop Biscuits	.	.	.	.	.	X	X	.	.	.	.	.	.	.
Cut Biscuits	.	.	.	.	.	X	X	.	.	.	.	.	.	.
BBP Biscuits	.	.	.	.	.	X	.	.	.	.	.	.	.	.
RBP Biscuits	.	.	.	.	.	.	.	.	.	.	.	.	.	.
Rye Muffins	.	.	.	.	.	.	.	.	.	.	.	.	.	.
Apple Muffins	.	.	.	.	.	X	.	.	.	.	X	.	.	.
Peach Muffins	.	.	.	.	.	X	.	.	.	.	X	.	.	.
Sweet Pineapple Muffins	.	.	.	.	.	X	.	.	.	.	X	.	.	.
Rice Muffins	.	.	.	.	.	X	.	.	.	.	X	.	.	.

BUT I CAN'T EAT THAT

RECIPE CHART

X means that ingredient is contained in the recipe.

A=CHEMICALS	F=EGG	K=CORN
B=ARTIFICIAL COLOR	G=YEAST	L=CHICKEN
C=CANE SUGAR	H=BEEF	M=TOMATOES
D=WHEAT	I=MALT OR BARLEY	N=POTATO
E=MILK	J=OATS	

```
                                  A B C D E F G H I J K L M N
BREADS
Corn Pone Pancakes               . . . . . . . . . . . . . X . . . . . .
Corn Bread                       . . . . . . . . . . . . . X . . . . . .
Zucchini Pancakes                . . . . . . . . . . . . . . . . . . . .
Zucchini Pancakes (Regular)      . . . . . X . . . X . . . . . . . . . .
Fresh Corn Pancakes              . . . . . . . . . X . . . . . X . . . .
Auntie's Pancakes                . . . . . X.X.X . . . . . . . . . . . .
Rice Pancakes                    . . . . . . . . . . . . . . . . . . . .
Orange Pancakes                  . . . . . X . . . X . . . . . . . . . .
Green Pancakes                   . . . . . . . . . . . . . . . . . . . .
DOUGHS
BASIC PASTA: Ravioli             . . . . . X . . . X . . . . . . . . . .
Vegetable Noodles                . . . . . X . . . X . . . . . . . . . .
Spinach, Beets, Carrots, Tomato  . . . . . X . . . X . . . . . . . . . .
Fried Noodles                    . . . . . X . . . X . . . . . . . . . .
Pastry Dough                     . . . . . X . . . . . . . . . . . . . .
Meat Turnovers                   . . . X.X . . . . . . . . . . . . . . .
Allergy Waffles                  . . . . . X . . . X . . . . . . . . . .
Blueberry or Fruit Waffles       . . . . . X . . . X . . . . . . . . . .
Carob Waffles                    . . . . . X . . . X . . . . . . . . . .
Carob Chip Waffles               . . . . . X . . . X . . . . . . . . . .
Chocolate Waffles                . . . . . X . . . X . . . . . . . . . .
Flour Tortillas                  . . . . . X . . . . . . . . . . . . . .
RICE
Basic White Rice                 . . . . . . . . . . . . . . . . . . . .
Basic Brown Rice                 . . . . . . . . . . . . . . . . . . . .
Crock Pot Brown Rice             . . . . . . . . . . . . . . . . . . . .
Ready Brown Rice                 . . . . . . . . . . . . . . . . . . . .
Herbs and Rice                   . . . . . . . . . . . . . . . . . . . .
Brown Rice Cakes                 . . . . . . . . . . . . . . . . . . . .
Fried "Rice A Tuna"              . . . . . . . . . . . . . . . . . . . .
Indian Wehani Rice               . . . . . . . . . . . . . . . . . . . .
Captain J.R.'s Seafood Specialty . . . . . . . . . . . . . . . . . . . .
Sweet Peach Breakfast Rice       . . . . . . . . . . . . . . . . . . . .
Apple Breakfast Delight          . . . . . . . . . . . . . . . . . . . .
```

BUT I CAN'T EAT THAT

RECIPE CHART
X means that ingredient is contained in the recipe.

A=CHEMICALS	F=EGG	K=CORN
B=ARTIFICIAL COLOR	G=YEAST	L=CHICKEN
C=CANE SUGAR	H=BEEF	M=TOMATOES
D=WHEAT	I=MALT OR BARLEY	N=POTATO
E=MILK	J=OATS	

```
                                         A B C D E F G H I J K L M N
FRUITS AND VEGETABLES
Apples                                   . . . . . . . . . . . . . .
Microwave Applesauce                     . . . . . . . . . . . . . .
Crockpot Applesauce                      . . . . . . . . . . . . . .
Applesauce                               . . . . . . . . . . . . . .
Applesauce Tips                          . . . . . . . . . . . . . .
Apple Smoothie                           . . . . . . . . . . . . . .
Simple Fruit Sauce                       . . . . . . . . . . . . . .
Quicker Sauces                           . . . . . . . . . . . . . .
Apple Butter                             . . . . . . . . . . . . . .
Jam Formula                              . . . . . . . . . . . . . .
Apple Jello                              . . . . . . . . . . . . . .
Apple Puff                               . . . . . . X . . . . . . .
Frozen Watermelon                        . . . . . . . . . . . . . .
Peach Butter                             . . . . . . . . . . . . . .
Fruit Ideas                              . . . . . . . . . . . . . .
CARROTS
Baked Shredded Carrots                   . . . . . . . . . . . . . .
Grated Carrot Salad                      . . . . . . . . . . . . . .
Carrot Sauce                             . . . . . . . . . . . . . .
Sweet Thins                              . . . . . . . . . . . . . .
CORN
Smashed Corn                             . . . . . . . . . . X . . .
Corn Pancakes                            . . . . . . X . . . X . . .
POTATOES
Potato Cakes                             . . . . . . X . . . . . . X
Potato Chips                             . . . . . . . . . . . . . X
Potato Croutons                          . . . . . . . . . . . . . X
Plain Baked Potatoes                     . . . . . . . . . . . . . X
Fries                                    . . . . . . . . . . . . . X
Skillet Hash Browns                      . . . . . . . . . . . . . X
ZUCCHINI
Broiled Zucchini                         . . . . . . . . . . . . . .
Zucchini Cakes                           . . . . . . X . . . . . . .
Microwaved Zucchini                      . . . . . . . . . . . . . .
Your Favorite Veggies                    . . . . . . . . . . . X . .
Stir Fry Bok Choy                        . . . . . . . . . . . X . .
Creamy Spinach                           . . . . . . . . . . . X . .
```

BUT I CAN'T EAT THAT

RECIPE CHART
X means that ingredient is contained in the recipe.

A=CHEMICALS	F=EGG	K=CORN
B=ARTIFICIAL COLOR	G=YEAST	L=CHICKEN
C=CANE SUGAR	H=BEEF	M=TOMATOES
D=WHEAT	I=MALT OR BARLEY	N=POTATO
E=MILK	J=OATS	

```
                                A B C D E F G H I J K L M N
```

CELERY IDEAS
Recipe	A B C D E F G H I J K L M N
Steamed, Microwaved, or Boiled Celery	. . . .
Celery Stuffing	. . . .
Herbal Vegetable Sauté	. . . .
Steaming Veggies Timetable	. . . .

SALAD IDEAS
Recipe	A B C D E F G H I J K L M N
Salad Dressing for Fruits	. . . .
Shredded Carrot Salad	. . . .
One Meal Salad	. . . . . . X . . . . . X . . .

SOUPS
Recipe	A B C D E F G H I J K L M N
BASIC: Chicken Stock	. . . . X . . .
BASIC: Beef Stock	. . . . X . . . . . .
BASIC: Lamb Stock	. . . .
BASIC: Vegetable Broth	. . . . X . X
Vegetable Broth Ideas	. . . .
Thicker Vegetable Soup	. . . .
Chunky Vegetable Soup	. . . .
Lite Lettuce Soup	. . . .
Cream of Lettuce Soup	. . . .
Quick Broccoli Soup	. . . .
Cream of Broccoli Soup	. . . .
Basic: Anything Goes Soup	. . . . . X . . . . . X . . . . X . X . X . X
Fish Broth	. . . .

(SOUPS) CHICKEN STOCK IDEAS
Recipe	A B C D E F G H I J K L M N
Cream of Chicken Soup	. . . . X . . .
Celery Soup	. . . . X . . .
Cream of Celery Soup	. . . . X . . .
Spinach Soup	. . . . X . . .
Cream of Spinach Soup	. . . . X . . .
Basic: Cauliflower Soup	. . . . X . . .
Zucchini Soup	. . . . X . . .
Basic: Sweet Pea Soup	. . . . X . . .
Imperial Green Soup	. . . . X . . .

SAUCES and SEASONINGS
Recipe	A B C D E F G H I J K L M N
Basic: Pan Drippings	. . . . X . . . . . X . . .
Beef Seasoning	. . . .
Chicken Seasoning	. . . .
Pizza Seasoning	. . . .
Vegetable Seasoning	. . . .
Fish Seasoning	. . . .

RECIPE CHART

X means that ingredient is contained in the recipe.

A=CHEMICALS	F=EGG	K=CORN
B=ARTIFICIAL COLOR	G=YEAST	L=CHICKEN
C=CANE SUGAR	H=BEEF	M=TOMATOES
D=WHEAT	I=MALT OR BARLEY	N=POTATO
E=MILK	J=OATS	

```
                                   A B C D E F G H I J K L M N
SEASONINGS
Herbal Butter                      . . . . . . . . . . . . . . . . . . . . . . . . . . . . .
Sesame Butter                      . . . . . . . . . . . . . . . . . . . . . . . . . . . . .
Herbal Salt                        . . . . . . . . . . . . . . . . . . . . . . . . . . . . .
Chive Sauce                        . . . . . . . . . . . . . . . . . . . . . . . . . . . . .
Peanut Butter Sauce                . . . . . . . . . . . . . . . . . . . . . . . . . . . . .
Peach Sauce                        . . . . . . . . . . . . . . . . . . . . . . . . . . . . .
Pear Sauce                         . . . . . . . . . . . . . . . . . . . . . . . . . . . . .
Allergy Spaghetti Sauce            . . . . . . . . . . . . . . X . . . . . . . . X . .
MISCELLANEOUS
Carrot Dressing                    . . . . . . . . . . . . . . . . . . . . . . . . . . . . .
Croutons                           . . . . . . X . . . . . X . . . . . . . . . . . . . .
Dragon Cookies                     . . . . X.X.X.X . . . . . . . X . . . . . . . .
Cornmeal Drops                     . . . . . . X . . . . . . . . . . . X.X . . . . . .
Basic Drinks                       . . . . . . . . . . . . . . . . . . . . . . . . . . . . .
Pop                                . . . . . . . . . . . . . . . . . . . . . . . . . . . . .
Fruit Shake                        . . . . . . . . . . . . . . . . . . . . . . . . . . . . .
Banana Dream Shake                 . . . . . . . . . . . . . . . . . . . . . . . . . . . . .
SWEET MEAL TOPPERS
Baked Whole Fruit                  . . . . . . . . . . . . . . . . . . . . . . . . . . . . .
BASIC: Apple Leather               . . . . . . . . . . . . . . . . . . . . . . . . . . . . .
Allergy Pie Pastry                 . . . . . . X . . . . . . . . . . . . . . . . . . . .
Allergy Apple Pie                  . . . . . . X . . . . . . . . . . . . . . . . . . . .
Allergy Strawberry Pie             . . . . . . X . . . . . . . . . . . . . . . . . . . .
Allergy Peach Pie                  . . . . . . X . . . . . . . . . . . . . . . . . . . .
Lite Allergy Pumpkin Pie           . . . . . . X . . . X . . . . . . . . . . . . . . .
Apple Envelope                     . . . . . . X . . . . . . . . . . . . . . . . . . . .
Allergy Angel Food Cake            . . . . . . X . . . X . . . . . . . . . . . . . . .
Customized Granola                 . . . . . . . . . . . . . . . . . . . . . X . . . . . .
Fructose Reduced Syrup             . . . . . . . . . . . . . . . . . . . . . . . . . . . . .
Allergy Pineapple Pudding          . . . . . . . . . . . . . . . . . . . . . . . . . . . . .
Lite Watermelon Freeze             . . . . . . . . . . . . . . . . . . . . . . . . . . . . .
Ultra Smooth Fruit Sauce           . . . . . . . . . . . . . . . . . . . . . . . . . . . . .
Breakfast Apple Fritters           . . . . . . X . . . X . . . . . . . . . . . . . . .
Allergy Pizzelles                  . . . . . . X . . . X . . . . . . . . . . . . . . .
Crisp Rice Treats                  . . . . . . . . . . . . . . . . . . . . . . . . . . . . .
Butterflies                        . . . . . . X . . . X . . . . . . . . . . . . . . .
Butter Cookies                     . . . . . . X.X . . . . . . . . . . . . . . . . . . .
Eatable Short Bread                . . . . . . X.X . . . . . . . . . . . . . . . . . . .
```

CHAPTER 1

INGREDIENTS AND SUBSTITUTIONS

FLOURS
For cake flour substitute one cup all purpose flour minus two tablespoons will equal one cup of cake flour. Sift both flours before measuring.

For one cup of wheat flour other ingredients can be used; 7/8 cup rice flour; 1 and 1/3 cup rolled oats; 1 cup Tapioca flour. IF: try 1/2 cup ground nuts.

For one tablespoon of wheat flour when using as a thickener, try 1/2 tablespoon Arrowroot; 1 egg; 1/2 tablespoon gelatin (non flavored); 1/2 tablespoon rice flour; 2 teaspoons Tapioca (instant); 1/2 tablespoon Tapioca flour; 2 tablespoons uncooked rice OR one tablespoon of Cream of Rice Cereal (OR other creamed cereals)

IF: 1 cup of wheat flour equals 1 and 1/4 cups of rye meal; 5/8 cups potato-starch flour; 3/4 cup cornmeal; 1/2 cup rye flour plus 1/2 cup potato flour; 5/8 cup rice flour plus 1/3 cup potato flour; 5/8 cup rice flour plus 1 and 1/3 cup rye flour. 1 tablespoon of wheat flour equals 1/2 tablespoon cornstarch; 1/2 tablespoon potato starch flour.

NOTE: When baking mixtures of other flours remember to cook for a longer time period at lower temperatures. Expect item to be crumbly in texture.

EGG
For one egg replacement there are different formulas to use. One egg equals: 1 teaspoon Arrowroot; 2 tablespoons water with 2 teaspoons baking powder; 1 1/2 tablespoons oil with 1 1/2 tablespoons of water with 1 teaspoon baking powder mixed together and added at one time. (I like this one the best) You can also use 3 tablespoons of a fruit puree; 1 teaspoon non flavored gelatin mixed with 2 tablespoons liquid (this is good for soups and fruits) OR 1/2 tablespoon lard with 1 tablespoon baking powder and 4 tablespoons apple sauce (OR flour).

BUT I CAN'T EAT THAT

CHAPTER 1

<u>INGREDIENTS AND SUBSTITUTIONS</u>

MILK

<u>Oat milk</u> substitute is made for use in cooking and on cereal. Mix one cup of water plus 2 teaspoons rolled oats, put into a blender and mix until smooth.

<u>Zucchini milk</u> You can cook with this milk and it freezes well. To get <u>white</u> zucchini milk, peel skin completely off. For <u>green</u> zucchini milk peal thinly. Chunk cut and use blender to liquefy. Heat to boil and scald (as in milk). Cool. Keep refrigerated for one week or freeze.

Use egg whites (using extra large eggs) for a <u>Milk</u> <u>substitute</u>, beat until foamy but not stiff.

        1 egg white = 1/2 - 1 cups milk
        2 egg whites = 1 1/2 - 2 cups milk
        3 egg whites = 2 1/2 - 3 cups milk.

When looking for a <u>milk</u> substitute in cookies, quick breads, pancakes, crepes or muffins, try 1 tablespoon lard plus fruit juice OR pureed vegetables OR fruits.

SUGAR

Many foods are good without sugar when fresh and prepared correctly. One of the best investments to achieve great flavor in foods, especially in vegetables, is a steamer. It assures minimum nutritional and vitamin loss.

<u>Sugar Substitute</u> using fructose in place of sugar, if tolerated. The following adjustments are 3/4 cup fructose to 1 cup of sugar and 2/3 teaspoon fructose to 1 teaspoon of sugar, if using fructose in <u>cold</u> beverages. One teaspoon fructose is equal to 1 teaspoon sugar in <u>hot</u> drinks. Six tablespoons fructose to 1/2 cup of sugar and 3/4 cup of fructose to 1 cup of sugar when <u>baking</u>.

<u>Fructose Reduced Syrup</u>
    1/2 cup fructose
    1/4 cup water

    Dissolve fructose in water. In a small sauce pan whisk mixture continuously on medium-high heat. Stir until mixture becomes syrupy and reaches the ball stage. (As in candy making, test a drop in cold water. If it balls up, it is ready.)

BUT I CAN'T EAT THAT

CHAPTER 1

INGREDIENTS AND SUBSTITUTIONS

EXTRA'S USED IN COOKING

To make your own corn and aluminum free <u>baking powder</u> sift together three times, store in a air tight container: 2 teaspoons cream of tartar, 2 teaspoons Arrowroot and 1 teaspoon baking soda. Use fresh ingredients and make baking powder frequently for best results.

When looking for a substitute for <u>bread crumbs</u> to add to meat mixtures try crushed rice cakes; rice krispies; Cream of Rice Cereal; grated carrots OR grated cauliflower.

For a <u>butter</u> replacement use clarified butter OR 7/8 cup Safflower oil plus 1/2 teaspoon salt to equal 1 cup of butter. Microwave 1 pound of butter, cut into 4 quarters. Heat on medium high until melted, watching. Skim top residue off and discard bottom residue. The clear middle liquid is now clarified. Cover. Do not refrigerate.

For 1 <u>fresh celery</u> stalk use celery salt: 1 to 2 teaspoons to taste.

For 1 <u>fresh onion</u> use onion power: 1 tablespoon for a small onion.

Use the <u>Vanilla Beans</u> for cooking then discarded when done or kept in your sweetener (sugar or fructose) or flour container.

CHAPTER 1
INGREDIENTS AND SUBSTITUTIONS

MISCELLANEOUS

For a natural <u>Antacid</u>; use 1/2 teaspoon of baking soda in a small glass of water.

<u>Non-Citric Mayo Spread</u> (use sparingly)
This also can be used as a binder.
2 egg yolks
3/4 cup Safflower oil
Add to taste:
1/4 teaspoon sea salt
1/4 teaspoon onion salt
1/8 teaspoon paprika
1/4 teaspoon celery salt
spices to add color – turmeric (yellow), dill and tarragon (green)

In the food processor blend egg yolks until light yellow. Add oil, drops at a time until it emulsifies. Add seasonings and salt. Do not expect this to taste like the store-bought mayonnaise.
IF: 1/4 teaspoon dried mustard

WATER
There's no substitution for the recommended daily 8 glasses of water daily to keep the body's systems functioning properly. It's no myth!

<u>TAP WATER</u> Extremely sensitive people may be bothered by the chemicals in everyday tap water. (Especially when traveling.) Boiling the tap water before drinking may help remove some of the impurities.

<u>SPRING WATER</u> is better than tap water, providing the extra minerals don't effect you. There is more sodium in spring water. Tap waters vary from city to city. (When traveling out of your city it is always wise to carry water with you, the water <u>you</u> have no reaction to.)

<u>DISTILLED WATER</u> is the closest you can get to pure no chemical, no mineral, sodium free water you can buy. It makes wonderful drinks, hot or cold. Test the different water sources for yourself to see which your body and taste buds prefer the most.
<u>FILTERED WATER</u>-Investigate installing a Reveres Osmosis Water Filter which pulls everything out of the water but the water!

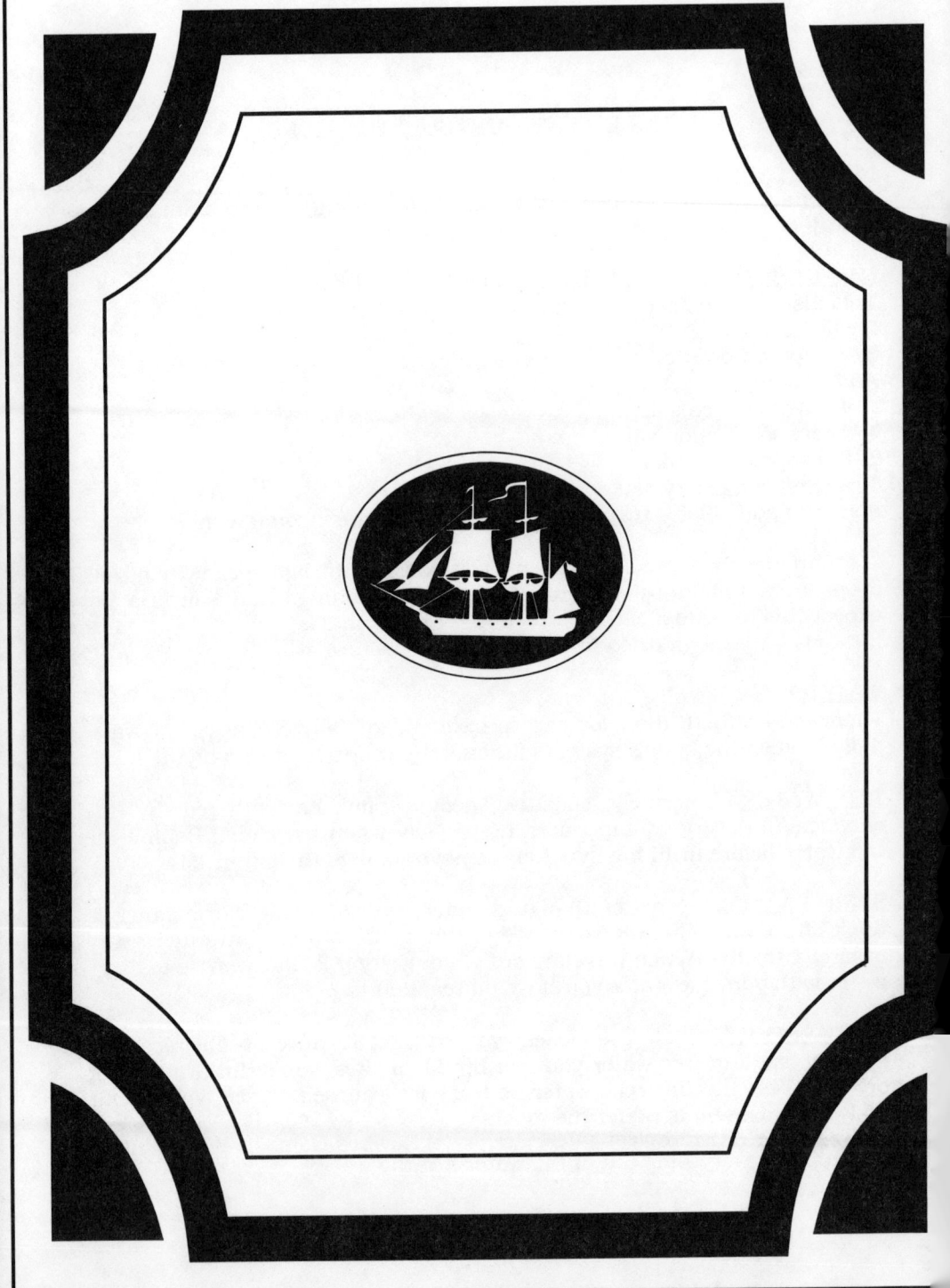

CHAPTER 1

TRAVEL

Avoiding allergens and additives in foods while traveling.

Eating while traveling presents problems for people with allergies. When traveling you must rely on phone books explicitly. Locating Health Food Stores in the area is helpful. Before going into any restaurant, call ahead to see what they will prepare that you can eat. Will they prepare vegetables steamed, meats unseasoned or items baked plain? Do the fries contain sulfates (many frozen potato products do) or are they made fresh on the premises. What ingredients lurk in their breading, MSG? What seasonings do they put in their hamburgers? Cover all your allergies. Only the chef of the establishment knows the correct answers to these questions. Make sure to speak to the right person. More restaurants are trying to accommodate patrons these days. Don't be afraid to send it back if it's not cooked as ordered. Bring your own oil and salt to the restaurant.

A small cooler is a good idea for carrying necessary basics and keeping freshly purchased foods cool. A small portable electric skillet is wonderful for reheating precooked rice and meat patties in your room. Pack as many carry on foods as possible, you will not know the availability and price of products along the way to your destination. Easy things to carry are; your special brand of crackers, cereals, water packed chicken, tuna or salmon, carrot sticks, rice chips, apples, etc. Bring cooked rice and only enough cooked meats for the 18 to 24 hour period (after which you hope to purchase fresh). You might be more willing to try this method when I say you will automatically come home feeling better and weighing less!

A good source of electrolytes are readily available in water solutions such as Pedilyte, Lytren Nursette and Ricelyte. These solutions are a "safe" item to have when traveling (and around the house at all times). Electrolytes works better than water to hydrate the body. It meets the body's requirement of potassium, phosphate, sodium, positive and negative ions to maintain the proper acid balance base you need. This balance is especially needed in illness, flu, heat and motion sickness by preventing dehydration and stabilizing the metabolism.

Distilled water from your home town would be a wise drink to bring along. Water is different outside your home area and is likely to upset your system.

Chapter 2

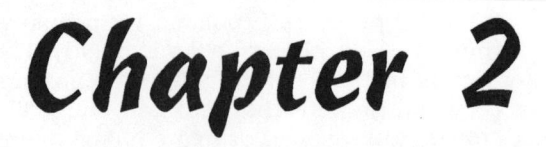

Proteins

Beef

Chicken

Eggs

Fish

Lamb, Pork, Veal

Miscellaneous

Peanut Butter, Turkey, Etc.

BUT I CAN'T EAT THAT

CHAPTER 2

BEEF CHOW MEIN
    2 pounds sirloin steak OR filet
    1 bag frozen sweet peas
    1/2 bag frozen snow pea pods
    1/2 teaspoon sea salt
    1/2 teaspoon ginger
    1 teaspoon fructose (optional)
    Napa cabbage
    Bok Choy
    1 tablespoon onion powder
    2 tablespoons Tapioca powder (OR Arrowroot)
    2 cups Beef Stock
    3-4 tablespoons Safflower oil
    Add water chestnuts, bean sprouts and bamboo shoots.

    Cut beef into 2"x1/4"x1/4" strips. Add oil to Wok. Heat to medium high. Cook vegetables, except peas and pods, for 10 minutes, stirring frequently. Remove from heat and cover to keep warm. Add more oil and sauté beef with seasonings until just cooked (slightly pink). Add thickener to Beef Stock then add meat, peas and pods. Stir until thickened. Add already cooked vegetables. Cook 1-2 minutes more. Serve over rice or fried homemade Pasta.

IF: Add 1-2 tablespoons each of oyster sauce and/or soy sauce. Optional, add 1 egg cooked omelet (sliced).

BUT I CAN'T EAT THAT

CHAPTER 2
EXTRA SAVORY MEAT LOAF
1 to 1 1/4 pounds combination meat loaf mix (beef and veal) OR (beef and pork) OR (beef, veal and pork)
3 tablespoons Cream of Rice OR Cream of Rye Cereal
3/4 cup cooked rice 1/2 cup bread crumbs or
1/2 cup allergy cereal (OR your favorite cereal)
1/3 cup water
1/2 cup finely chopped celery (sauté)
3 tablespoons parsley
1 tablespoon onion powder
1/4 tablespoon each, thyme, marjon, paprika, celery salt, savory and sweet basil
1/2 teaspoon sea salt
1 egg substitute (1/2 tablespoon oil, 1 1/2 tablespoon water mixed with 1 teaspoon homemade baking powder)

Mix all ingredients together thoroughly (by hand with a light touch). Line a 3"x10"x4" bread tin with wax paper. Put meat into the bread tin. Invert tin onto a rack and remove the wax paper. (If using ground sirloin beef and veal, do not use wax paper and cook in the tin.) Bake in a preheated 350 degree oven. If cooking a mixture with <u>pork included</u>, bake loaf for 1 hour 20 to 25 minutes. If cooking a mixture <u>without pork</u> bake loaf for 1 hour. Juices running out of the loaf when pierced should be clear when loaf is done. If the juices have a pink tinge, bake loaf 15-20 minutes longer. Loaf will look very browned. Serve hot or cold. Slice for lunches or freeze. Reheats nicely in the microwave.

IDEAS: Add grated cooked carrots OR grated cooked cauliflower (sauté) to raw meat mixture.
Sprinkle top of loaf with red paprika before cooking.
Freeze raw meat mixture for cooking later.
Can make hamburger patties out of all meat loaf mixtures.

IF: Substitute mashed potatoes OR oatmeal for rice cereal.
Serve hot with melted cheese (American or Colby) or over the top with a hot cheese sauce.
Use one real egg instead of the egg substitute.
Use evaporated milk OR tomato sauce for liquid.

PORCUPINE BALLS
1 recipe Extra Savory Meat Loaf (all beef)
Add 1/2 cup cooked brown rice.

Mix meat and rice together. Using a meat ball scooper, shape mixture into smoother balls with the palm of your hand. Bake 400 degrees for 20 minutes on a raised rack. Serve plain or in Allergy Spaghetti Sauce.

BUT I CAN'T EAT THAT

CHAPTER 2

HEIDI'S ALLERGY POT ROAST
    This recipe materialized because of my husband, Richard's, Boy Scouting escapades. He was a Scoutmaster who often camped and cooked two to three days in the wilderness. He asked me to buy "budget" meat for roasting on his outings. He cooked it himself with the Troop's heavy cast iron outdoor Dutch Oven. He and the other dads always came home bragging how good his dinners were. I finally had to try out this cooking pot. It answered all my problems of tough, dry, "budget" meat! It made the meat delicious. Now I think every kitchen should have a pot like that.

    4-5 pounds beef pot roast, blade, arm, English cut, brisket, bottom round, rump roast or eye of round
    3 celery stalks, chopped
    1/2 cup Beef Stock
    3/4 tablespoon paprika
    1/2 tablespoon thyme
    1 tablespoon onion salt
    lard (no preservative)

    Rub spices into the roast. In a heavy iron skillet melt lard and brown all sides of the roast. Discard lard and add stock to pan removing the solidified juices and pan drippings from the bottom. Layer the celery on the bottom of the heavy cast iron Dutch Oven. Place the roast on top of the celery. Pour stock over top. Cook in a preheated 300 degree oven for 3 hours until the meat pokes easily with a fork and falls apart. Drain juices and refrigerate. Remove the fats that forms on top of the juices. This roast is even better the next day.
*Use Arrowroot to thicken juices, adding sea salt to taste.

QUICK COOKING IDEAS:
    To make a roast in the <u>pressure cooker</u> use 1 1/2 cups of stock. Bring the stock to a boil then cap. Reduce heat, letting cap rock. Cook for 35 minutes. Remove pressure cooker from heat. Let pressure drop on it's own accord.

CHAPTER 2

SWISS STEAK
    1 1/2 inch thick round steak
    1/2 teaspoons onion powder
    1/4 teaspoons paprika
    1/2 teaspoon Bouquet Garni
    1-1 1/2 cups Beef Stock
    1 carrot (sliced)
    1 1/2 tablespoon Arrowroot or more if needed, mixed
    with equal amounts of cold water OR stock
    2 large tomatoes (peeled and seeded)

Poke steak all over with a fork on both sides before browning to tenderize. Rub spices into steak. In a heavy skillet melt lard for browning. Brown all sides of the steak. Discard lard. Add the stock to the pan removing the solidified juices and pan drippings from the bottom with a fork. Place steak on the bottom of a heavy Dutch Oven. Pour stock over top. Add tomatoes and carrots. Cook in a preheated 300 degree oven for 3 hours until meat pokes easily with fork and falls apart. Drain stock juices and refrigerate. Remove solid fats from the top. (When cooking Swiss Steak on a burner, meat needs 1 hour cooking time until fork comes out easily.) When done, use the food processor to smoothly blend the stock, tomatoes and carrots. Thicken juices for gravy with Arrowroot.

IDEAS: More carrots can be added for additional sweetness. Use V-8 juice for liquid to give Swiss Steak a tangier flavor.
Add a 16 oz. canned of diced tomatoes, instead of fresh, before cooking round steak.

QUICK COOKING IDEAS:
    To make Swiss Steak in a <u>pressure cooker</u>, use 1 cup of stock with steak. Bring the stock to a boil then cap. Reduce heat, letting cap rock for 15 minutes. Remove pressure cooker from heat. Let the pressure drop on it's own accord.

BUT I CAN'T EAT THAT

CHAPTER 2

<u>BEEF STEW</u>
    2 to 3 pounds cubed beef (1"inch)
    1/2 cups Tapioca flour
    2-3 celery stalks with leafs, chopped
    2 small carrots, sliced
    1 tablespoon onion powder
    1/2 teaspoon Bouquet Garni
    2 Bay leaves
    1/4 teaspoon paprika
    1/4 teaspoon sea salt
    2 cups Beef Stock
    2-3 tablespoons lard (no preservative) for browning
    Bones; calf or beef feet

Place 1/3-1/2 cup Tapioca flour in a plastic bag with all seasonings. Shake meat in bag to coat. In a heavy iron skillet melt lard for browning. Brown meat pieces. Discard lard. Make a bed of chopped celery on bottom of the same skillet. Add meat and Bay leaves. Add stock to meat. Cook with calf or beef feet for extra flavor. Cover tightly with lid or aluminum foil. Bring stock to boil, reduce to low, cook for 1 hour. Add vegetables during the last half hour. Bring liquid up to a boil again when adding vegetables. Then reduce heat and continue cooking for remainder of time. Remove bones and bay leaves. Serve over top of hot rice. Garnish with parsley.

IDEAS: Add other spices IE., garlic powder.
              Add sweet peas OR green beans.
              Lamb OR Veal may be used with their own stocks.
              Cuts that can be used:
                      Beef: chunk, round or rump
                      Lamb: shoulder cuts
                      Veal: ribs, loin, shoulder cuts
IF: Potatoes can be added with veggies in the last half hour.

QUICK COOKING IDEAS:
    To make Beef Stew in a <u>pressure cooker</u> use 1 cup of stock. Bring the stock to a boil then cap. Reduce heat, letting cap rock. Cook for 10 minutes. Remove cooker from heat and then cool quickly.

CHAPTER 2

<u>S.O.M. MORE</u> (Save Our Mouth)
A great allergy dish for people with orthodonture work or newly placed or adjusted braces.
- 1 to 2 pounds of cubed beef stew meat (browning meat is optional)
- 1/2 cup water
- 1-2 Bay leaves
- 1 teaspoon celery salt
- 1/4 teaspoon paprika
- 2 tablespoons Arrowroot
- Cream of Brown Rice Cereal

Before going to bed add cubed beef to Crock Pot with the rest of the ingredients except Rice Cereal. Cook overnight on low 10-11 hours. In the morning separate the liquid the from the meat and store in refrigerator, discarding Bay leaves.

At supper time remove fat from the liquid. Whisk cold liquid with 2 tablespoons of Arrowroot and place into a small pan. Heat liquid up slowly to thicken, stirring often. (Careful not to boil.) As liquid thickens it becomes clear. Remove from heat immediately.

In a food processor loosely chop 1/2 of the cooked meat to resemble ground meat. Add this to the hot liquid and pour over prepared Cream of Brown Rice Cereal (prepare as per directions on box). Season with sea salt to taste. Serve remaining stew to others as a chunky stew.

TO MICROWAVE LIQUID: Cook 1 1/2 minutes on 80 % power. Stir. Microwave 1 minute on 70.% power. Stir. Microwave 1 minute on 80% power. Stir. You may need 50 seconds more on 80% power again.

IDEAS: Serve over rice, rice macaroni, mashed potatoes OR in a puff pastry shell.
Add cooked celery, carrots, peas, potatoes or other tolerated vegetables.

CHAPTER 2
LEFTOVER BEEF PIE
    2-3 cups leftover beef stew OR roast meat
    1 1/2 cups Beef Stock
    1 1/2 tablespoon Arrowroot
    1 cup leftover veggies
    1 Allergy Pie Pastry
    sea salt to taste

Cut leftover meat into bite sized pieces. For people with <u>mold allergy use meat that is not more than 18 hours old</u>. Use meat that has been frozen <u>before</u> this period. Whisk Arrowroot and cold stock together. Season with sea salt. In a casserole or deep dish pie pan add leftover stock to meat. Mix in leftover carrots, sweet peas, green beans, corn or any vegetable desired. Cover with leftover or extra pie crust. Slit top in several places. Bake 425 degrees for about 15-20 minutes. Great quick meal.

IDEAS: Precook pastry top on parchment paper, on a cookie sheet. (Preheat oven to 425 degrees, bake for 8-10 minutes.)
*For a quicker cooking time, thicken cold stock with Arrowroot over medium high heat, stirring constantly. Stock will become clear. Do not over cook. Combine all meat and veggies when sauce is hot. Add precooked top to cover.

IF: Serve with biscuits on top instead of pie crust.
Diced baked potatoes are good to add.
Brush crust with leftover eggs, yolks or whites
    for nicer browning.

FLANK STEAK
    2 pounds Flank steak or 4 thin Roulades
    1 cup Celery Stuffing
    1/2 teaspoon paprika
    1 tablespoon cold water
    1 tablespoon Arrowroot

Rub paprika liberally on the outside of the Flank steak. Work spice in well. Score the outside of the meat only. Stuff meat with 2-3 tablespoons of Celery Stuffing and roll. Place in Crock Pot (no water). Cook covered for 6 to 10 hours. Meat will be beautifully browned. Make gravy out of juices by whisking cold water with the Arrowroot. Add to hot juices stirring constantly over medium high heat. Gravy will become clear. Do not boil. Spoon over the top of the meat OR offer on the side.
*The scoring makes this a very attractive dish.

BUT I CAN'T EAT THAT

CHAPTER 2

HAMBURGER

Everyone disagrees on which ground hamburger meat has the best flavor. It depends on the individuals taste which cut of beef to use. Sirloin, round or chuck? Hamburger meat is really best when you grind it fresh yourself. Sirloin needs a little Safflower oil in the pan to keep it from sticking. Chuck needs to have the fat drained along the way while cooking. Round is in between. Handle this meat gently and the outcome will be juicier. You do need to use more pressure when making hamburgers for the grill so the meat is firm enough to stay on top of the grill!

    1/4 pound of freshly ground beef (your choice)
    1 preheated cast iron skillet
    sprinkle pan with sea salt (optional)
    sprinkle pan with Safflower oil (optional)

Prepare a skillet with oil and salt. Using sea salt in the frying pan before adding the meat helps with extra browning, plus gives added flavor. Preheat pan on medium high heat. Place hamburger patty in the middle of the skillet. Cover with a splatter screen. Do not use a solid lid. Cook until the blood raises to top of the patty and the bottom is browned, 5-7 minutes. Flip the hamburger over and cook until the blood rises to top of the patty, for 4 more minutes. Remove immediately. There is nothing worse than a tough, dry "over-cooked" burger.

IDEAS:
    Timing is less for thinner patties and more for thicker patties.
    You may want to turn the heat down to medium after both sides are browned.
    For thicker patties the middle of the hamburger may be stuffed.
    Use this recipe with all Allergy Meatloaf mix combinations.
    Burgers are great with thickened pan drippings, meat juices OR broth over top.
    Grill over charcoal (No gas grilling OR lighterfluid. Use an electric starter when possible to avoid allergy reactions.)

IF: Melt cheese over top of hamburgers during the last 2 minutes.
    Blue cheese with green olives stuffed in middle of a hamburger is wonderfully tasty, your guests will love them.
    Golden mushroom soup is great over top of hamburgers for a Salisbury steak dinner.

CHAPTER 2

HAMBURGER SKILLET TOSS
    1 pound of ground beef sirloin
    1 tablespoon onion powder
    1/4-1/2 teaspoon each: sweet basil, thyme, marjoram, and savory
    1/2 cup celery, minced
    sea salt to taste
    1-2 cups cooked brown rice
    2 tablespoons Safflower oil

    Basic: Brown ground beef, breaking it into small pieces. Add spices and set aside. In the meat juices left in the pan sauté minced celery 5-10 minutes. Add cooked rice and season with sea salt to taste. Sauté. If needed, add 1-2 tablespoons Safflower oil. Mix all ingredients and heat thoroughly. Garnish with parsley flakes OR fresh chives.

IDEAS: Add color to dish with turmeric (yellow) OR paprika (red)
            Add any meats, poultry, or fish
            Add poultry seasoning to chicken
            Add curry seasoning to lamb
            Add any vegetables that are tolerated
            Use cut fruits and omit the seasonings
            Substitute shredded zucchini for rice (drain first)
            Use homemade pasta instead of rice
            Add gravy and serve over toasted rice bread
            Use your own combo of spices
IF: As extras use: cheese, bean sprouts, beans, mushrooms, garlic, sherry, diced tomatoes OR lemons.

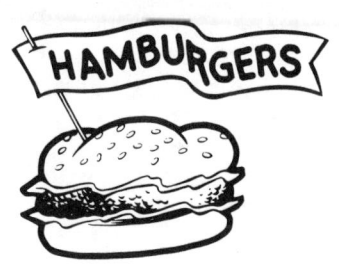

BUT I CAN'T EAT THAT

CHAPTER 2

<u>HAMBURGER BAKE</u>
   1 pound ground beef round
   1 tablespoon onion powder
   1/4 teaspoon garlic powder
   1 pound elbow macaroni made with brown rice flour
   2-2 1/2 cups Allergy Spaghetti Sauce

Brown the ground beef with onion and garlic powder. Drain. Cook macaroni per instructions on box. (You can use shell macaroni made with brown rice flour.) Drain. Mix beef and macaroni with sauce. Put into a casserole dish and bake in a preheated 350 degree oven for 20-25 minutes.

IDEAS: Use thickened Beef Stock if tomatoes can not be tolerated.
IF: Sprinkle Parmesan cheese over top.
         Add 1/2 cup cottage cheese to mixture before putting into casserole.
         Mix 1/2 cup shredded mozzarella cheese to mixture before putting in casserole.

<u>Quick Beef Meal Ideas</u>
   Steak-Ums, leftover roast OR ground beef
   Allergy Spaghetti Sauce
   shredded lettuce
   shredded carrots
   shredded zucchini
   diced tomatoes
   Homemade Burritos or Tortillas (Use regular or rye)

Store bought Steak-Ums are safe and fast for stuffing Burritos or Tortillas. Slice up leftover roast OR cooked ground beef. Spoon 1-2 tablespoons of sauce over the meat. Heat in the microwave 30-50 seconds on 80% power. Top with shredded lettuce, carrots, and zucchini. Roll up and enjoy.

IF: Sprinkle cheese over the top of the meat before microwaving.

CHAPTER 2

MEAT STUFFED ZUCCHINI
>   large zucchini for stuffing
>   1 pound ground meat OR poultry
>   1/2 teaspoon sea salt
>   1 tablespoon onion powder
>   1/4 teaspoon thyme
>   1/4 teaspoon poultry seasoning for poultry
>   1/4 teaspoon marjoram for lamb
>   1/4 cup parsley
>   3/4 cup cooked brown rice
>   1 extra zucchini shredded

Cut large zucchini in half and scoop out the center seeds and steam for 5-7 minutes. Drain and dry. OR boil whole zucchini in water for 10 minutes. When cool, cut in half. Scoop out the center seeds, invert on paper toweling and drain. Sauté meats with seasonings. Remove from the pan and drain. Mix the rice with the meat mixture. Sauté the shredded zucchini 5-7 minutes and drain. Mix with rice and meat OR use shredded zucchini as a topping over the stuffed meat. Stuff zucchini and bake in a preheated 400 degree oven for 20 minutes or until browned.

IDEAS: Use Allergy Spaghetti Sauce with meat, spooning sauce over top of meat mixture before cooking.
Sprinkle paprika over top.
Add more spices, jazzing it up to suit your own taste.
Substitute bread crumbs for rice.

IF: Melt mozzarella cheese over the top of the stuffing during the last 5 minutes.

CHAPTER 2

<u>PUREED MEAT</u>
For stuffing ravioli, meat pies or snacks on rye or rice crackers. Good for finger sandwiches.
    1 hamburger patty (1/4 pound)
    1 veal patty (1/4 pound)
    1/2 teaspoon onion powder
    1/4 teaspoon paprika
    1/4 teaspoon celery salt
    1/4 teaspoon sea salt
    1-2 teaspoons Safflower oil OR broth
    1 teaspoon fresh chopped chives
    sprinkle of savory

Cook all ingredients except oil (OR broth). Drain. Transfer to food processor and puree until meat starts looking like mud and sticks to the sides. Add liquids, small amounts at a time with machine running. You do not want the mixture to be to thin. It should really stick to your spoon, but be soft enough to spread.

IDEAS: This makes a great high protein snack!
IF: Substitute an egg for the Safflower oil.

CHAPTER 2

ALL HOMEMADE LASAGNA
1 recipe of Basic: Lasagna Pasta
1 1/2 to 2 pounds meat loaf mix (Butcher's combo, ground pork and beef)
3 1/2 cups Allergy Spaghetti Sauce
1 pound mozzarella cheese (shredded)
1-2 eggs
2 cups or 1 pound dry cottage cheese
1/2-3/4 cup grated Parmesan cheese

Cook meat and drain well. Heat sauce for easy spreading. Cook noodles and lay on (oiled) wax paper. Use a 13x9 inch rectangle pan. Add some sauce to the bottom of the pan before starting layers. Start lining pan bottom with noodles laying them side by side. Add a layer of crumbled cooked meat, then place a layer of sauce over top of that. Mix the dry cottage cheese with the eggs. Spread 1/2 of the dry cottage cheese mix in a thin layer over the top of the sauce. Next, layer 1/2 of the mozzarella cheese over the top of the cottage cheese layer, sprinkling with 1/2 of the Parmesan cheese over top of that. Repeat this whole procedure one more time. Cook in a 375 degree preheated oven for 45 to 70 minutes. (Cooking time depends on how cold the dish is. Is it at room temperature before cooking?) Sauce should be bubbling when Lasagna is done cooking. Let Lasagna rest 10 minutes before cutting.

IDEAS: Freeze in individual portions for wonderful quick meals.
To heat up one piece – Microwave covered on a plate for 9 minutes at 50 % power. Then cook 1-2 minutes uncovered on 100 % power. Let stand 5 minutes.

CHAPTER 2

ALLERGY LASAGNA (No wheat, no cheese)
    3 large zucchini
    1 tablespoon Safflower oil
    16 ounces, Allergy Spaghetti sauce, cooked and ready
    1 pound fresh spinach chopped (OR frozen bag of chopped spinach with water squeezed out of it) cooked and ready
    pinch of nutmeg
    1/2 pound ground lamb
    1/4 cup cooked brown rice with the following added:
        1 tablespoon Safflower oil
        1/2 teaspoon dried oregano
        1/2 teaspoon dried basil
        1/2 teaspoon onion powder
        pinch of garlic powder (optional)

    Sauté rice in oil with all seasonings except nutmeg, until crispy. Set aside. Wash zucchini thoroughly. Trim ends off. Cut in thin slices. (Easy if you have a meat slicer.) Cut slabs 1/4 inch thick. Coat the front and back of zucchini slices with oil.
    Cook and drain lamb. Crumble lamb when cool. Add nutmeg to chopped spinach.
    Oil an 8"inch square baking dish. Place a layer of zucchini, then sauce, then 1/2 half spinach, then 1/2 of lamb. Repeat. Top with shredded zucchini. Sprinkle with toasted rice.
    Cook in a preheated 350 degree oven for 40 minutes or until top is browned and sauce is bubbly. (Add 15-20 minutes if dish is cold from the refrigerator). Lasagna freezes well.

IDEAS: To serve more people double the recipe and use a 9x13 inch baking dish.
            To heat up one piece of lasagna: Microwave covered on a microwavable plate for 9 minutes at 50 % power. Cook 1-2 minutes uncovered on 100 % power. Let stand 5 minutes.
IF: Use real onion and real garlic.
            Use canned sauces.

BUT I CAN'T EAT THAT

CHAPTER 2

CHICKEN

I have one thing to say about this. Chicken is not foul!

Chicken is the catchall of all meats. Its mild flavor and tenderness lends it to many dishes. Try substituting chicken in some of your best recipes. Buy the freshest chicken for best flavor and texture. The largest breasts make good roasts to slice up for sandwiches. Smaller breasts tend to be juicier and more tender. These are great to sauté and poach. Whether you camouflage it in a casserole or serve it plain, chicken is an excellent source of protein.

PLAIN BAKED CHICKEN
Rinse chicken breasts well. Drip dry. Place in a pan with a rack. Preheat oven to 350 degrees. Bake 1 hour. Chicken skins will brown and puff up crispy. For extra crispy skins sprinkle with salt before cooking.

PLAIN OVEN FRIED CHICKEN
Rinse chicken breasts well. Drain. Place on a T-Fal cookie sheet with a rim, skin side down. Preheat oven to 350 degrees. Bake for 1 hour. Chicken will self fry in its own oils. Season skins before cooking.

PLAIN MICROWAVED CHICKEN
Rinse chicken breasts well. Put chicken in a 9x13 inch glass casserole pan. Place 6 chicken breasts (2 pounds), skin can be off or on, side up with the thickest meaty side towards the outside of the pan. Cover with wax paper. If you have a revolving plate in the microwave, cook on 100% power for 12 minutes. (Rotate plate half way through cooking time if not.) Let stand covered in oven 5 minutes more. This method is also good for making chicken for soups. It keeps the chicken moist.
　*Use this method minus 4 minutes when grilling, barbecuing, OR boiling. You may want to brush with Safflower oil and add spices before barbecuing. This method browns the chicken and you are confident its cooked thoroughly.

Other menu plans can easily be generated to suit your taste buds, time frame and nutritional standards. Here are some combinations to get you started.

Breakfast
Allergy Sausage Patties
Rice Muffins

Snack
Zucchini Cakes

Lunch
Seafood Pilaf
Imperial Green Soup

Snack
Fresh Fruit w/
Salad Dressing for Fruits
Homemade Bread Sticks dipped
in Homemade Peanut Butter

Dinner
Marinated Chicken Breasts
Smashed Corn
Herbal Rice
Allergy Pizzels

Snack
Allergy Meat Loaf slices

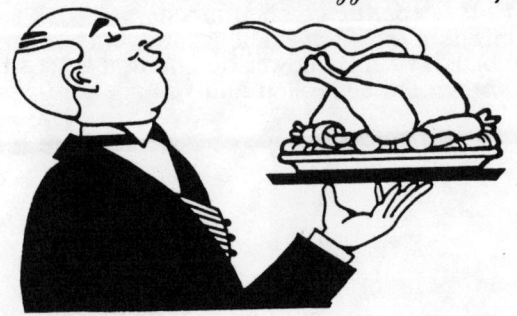

CHAPTER 2

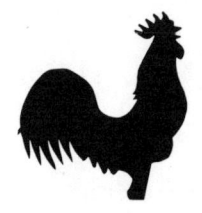

CROCK POT CHICKEN
Always rinse well and dry chicken before cooking.

1) <u>Roast</u> with chicken bones against the walls of Crock Pot. Cover and cook low 5 to 5 1/2 hours.

2) <u>Poached</u> chicken. Put meaty chicken pieces on the bottom of a Crock Pot first. Add Chicken Stock OR water to cover 1/2 way up the wall of the Crock Pot. Cover and cook on low for 5 to 5 1/2 hours.

3) <u>Browned</u> chicken. Brown with lard OR Safflower oil in a heavy skillet on medium high heat. Place in crock pot. Cover. Cook on low 5 to 5 1/2 hours.

4) <u>Not Browned</u>. Place chicken pieces flat on top of each other in a Crock Pot. Cook on <u>low</u> 5 1/2-6 hours, on <u>high</u> cook for 2 1/4 to 2 3/4 hours. (When cooking chicken on high heat, put carrot slices between the chicken and the sides of walls.)

CHAPTER 2

MARINATED CHICKEN BREASTS
    4 chicken breasts
    1/3 cup Safflower oil
    1/4 teaspoon each; sea salt, paprika, curry, marjoram,
    onion powder OR garlic powder, parsley and poultry
    seasoning.

Soak chicken in cold water 2 hours prior to marinating, in the refrigerator to prevent Salmonella poisoning. Pat dry. Mix in a plastic bag, Safflower oil with above seasonings OR your choice of them. Add the chicken and close the bag placing it on a plate in case it leaks. Flip bag over, on and off all day. Preheat oven to 350 degrees. Cook 1 hour covered with aluminum foil for the first 1/2 hour then uncover for the second 1/2 hour. Broil with skin side up for 5 minutes to crisp.

IF: Add to marinade sauce: soy sauce and honey
                              : lemon and/or tomato sauce
                              : V-8

*It's a good idea to learn how to bone your own chicken. It's easy and economical boning the chicken breasts yourself. Here are some ideas for boneless chicken.

NO FUSS CHICKEN DINNER
    3 pounds boneless chicken breasts
    3 carrots, peeled, sliced or diced
    3 celery stalks, diced
    1 tablespoon onion powder
    1/2 cup Chicken Stock
    1/4 teaspoon Bouquet Garni
    1/4 teaspoon poultry seasoning
    1/4-1/2 teaspoon sea salt
    2 tablespoons Arrowroot

Place celery and carrots on bottom of a Crock Pot. Cut all chicken, but two pieces, into bite size pieces and place on top of veggies. Add Chicken Stock and seasonings. Place two uncut pieces of chicken over top. Cover with the lid and cook on low 5 to 6 hours. Remove liquid. Mix Arrowroot in cold water and slowly whisk it into the hot (reserved) liquid. This thickens instantly from the heat of the liquid. Pour over chicken when serving. No Fuss Chicken Dinner keeps warm in the Crock Pot on low without over cooking.

BUT I CAN'T EAT THAT

CHAPTER 2

QUICK CHICKEN
With flat side of the meat hammer pound boneless chicken breasts flat. (Pound between two pieces of heavy upholstery plastic for easier handling.) You may do this beforehand, keeping it covered in a refrigerator or freeze until you need it.

Quick-broil chicken in oven 2 minutes per side. Top with Herbal Butter.

HOT CHICKEN SALAD
4 chicken breasts (boneless)
1 (16 oz.) can of cling peaches (in its own juice)
1/2 teaspoon ground ginger
Bib or Boston Lettuce
shredded iceberg lettuce
2 celery stalks (thinly sliced)
1 tablespoon Arrowroot

Cut into strips or cube 4 cooked boneless chicken breasts. Drain juice from peaches. Use peach juice with ginger as a marinade for the chicken. Refrigerate 5 hours or overnight, if using all of the chicken the next day. (A precaution to remember for people with mold allergies.) Put large Bib or Boston leaves on bottom of the platter then shredded Iceberg lettuce arrange as a nest to place chicken in.

Place celery slices in a ring on top of lettuce for design. Drain chicken, using peach juice mixed with Arrowroot, heating over medium heat until thick. Do not boil. Dice peaches. Add peaches and chicken to hot thickened juice. Serve in lettuce nest.

ONE STEP CHICKEN AND RICE
2 boneless chicken filets
1/2 cup Kloyco Rose rice
1/2 cup Sweet Rice
1 3/4 cup Chicken Stock
1/4 cup clarified butter OR Safflower oil
sea salt to taste

Mix Kloyco Rose with the Sweet Rice. Place 2 chicken filets on top of rice adding the Chicken Stock. Drizzle 1/4 cup clarified butter (OR Safflower oil) over chicken. Season with sea salt. Cover. Bake in a preheated 350 degree oven for 45-60 minutes. Serve hot.

BUT I CAN'T EAT THAT

CHAPTER 2

<u>CHICKEN POT PIE</u>
    3 cups uncooked diced chicken (OR turkey)
    1 (10 ounce) package frozen peas and carrots
    1 to 1 1/2 cups Chicken Stock
    1 pastry top with chicken cutouts for decoration
    1/2-2 tablespoons Tapioca flour

Combine Tapioca flour with stock. Mix in chicken and vegetables together. Cover with pastry top, pinch edges together tightly. Paste pastry cutouts on with water. Prick top before cooking allowing steam to escape. Bake in a preheated 350 degree oven for 45 minutes until bubbly.

IDEAS: For quicker cooking time:
    Precook pastry top on parchment paper on cookie sheet at preheated 425 degrees for 8-10 minutes until browned.
    Thicken cold broth with Arrowroot over medium high heat, stirring constantly. When broth becomes hot, add precooked pastry top to cover and serve.
IF: Brush with egg white wash over pastry for quicker browning.

<u>PASTRY TOP</u> (Makes two tops)
    2 cups all purpose flour
    1 teaspoon homemade baking powder
    1 teaspoon salt sense
    1/2 cup lard (check for no preservatives)
    OR 1/4 cup lard and 1/4 cup butter
    1/2 cup cold water (+1 tablespoon if to dry)

With a wire whisk blend flour, salt, and baking powder. Cut in lard with pastry cutter (OR two knives) until mix resembles the size of small peas. With a fork, gently mix water in, making a crumbly dough. Do not over work. If too dry, add 1 tablespoon of water at a time as needed. Cut dough in half. Roll out dough between two sheets of wax paper. Freeze extra crust.

BUT I CAN'T EAT THAT

CHAPTER 2

BREADED CHICKEN STRIPS
    1 1/2 to 2 pounds boneless chicken breasts, cut into 1 inch strips (pound to even out breasts)
    1 egg, beaten
    1 cup homemade bread crumbs
    1/4 teaspoon paprika
    1/4 teaspoon poultry seasoning
    Tapioca flour OR Rice flour
    1/2 cup Safflower oil OR clarified butter

First, dust chicken with flour. Then dip chicken into the beaten egg. Mix bread crumbs with paprika and poultry seasoning and bread chicken strips. Refrigerate for one half hour to set. Pour oil in a T-Fal baking sheet with a lip and place pan in a preheated 375 degree oven. Preheat 10-15 minutes. Add chicken strips, turning to coat both sides of strips. Cook 30-40 minutes until brown and crispy.

CHICKEN AND TOMATO CASSEROLE
    1 1/2 cups cooked Basic Pasta OR Vegetable Noodles
    1 to 2 cups cooked diced chicken
    1 cup Allergy Spaghetti Sauce
    1/2 teaspoon sweet basil

In a small casserole put a thin layer of noodles, then a layer of chicken. Pour 1/2 cup sauce over top. Layer noodles and chicken pouring remainder of sauce over top. Sprinkle with basil. Bake uncovered in a preheated 350 degree oven for 25 minutes.

IF: Sprinkle Parmesan and mozzarella cheese in between layers and on top.
    Sprinkle top with parsley and black olives.
    Use rice instead of noodles.
    Instead of tomato sauce: Use Cream Sauce made with milk OR Chicken Stock, dot with butter then top with crumbled potato chips.

BUT I CAN'T EAT THAT

CHAPTER 2
ALLERGY CHICKEN CHOW MEIN
    2 1/2 pounds boneless chicken filets, cut 1/2 inch squares OR strips
    1/2 teaspoon ground ginger
    1 tablespoon onion powder
    2 tablespoons Safflower oil (or more if needed)
    3 celery stalks, sliced
    1 1/2 cups Bok Choy, sliced
    1/2-1 teaspoon sea salt
    1 1/4 cup Chicken Stock with 1 tablespoon Tapioca flour
    1/2 cup cooked carrots

Add oil to Wok and heat on medium high heat. Sauté chicken with all spices, stirring constantly. Remove and keep warm. Add more oil to the Wok and sauté vegetables, except carrots, until done (5 minutes). Add Chicken Stock with flour, stir until thick. Add chicken and carrots last. Serve over fried Pasta OR rice.

IDEA: Add water chestnuts, bean sprouts, and bamboo shoots.
IF: For people with no mold allergies, add soy sauce.

CHICKEN AND RICE SCRAPPLE
    1 cup Chicken Stock
    1/4 cup minced celery
    1/2 teaspoon savory
    1 tablespoon onion powder
    1 1/2 tablespoon Arrowroot
    2 tablespoons parsley
    1 tablespoon Safflower oil
    1 cup cooked long grain rice
    1 1/2 cups cooked chicken, finely diced
    Tapioca flour

In the food processor fine chop the chicken. Add the rice and process 3-4 pulses getting an even mixture. Sauté celery in oil. In a saucepan mix spices and Arrowroot together with stock. Heat on medium high heat until stock thickens. Add rice and chicken stirring constantly for 1/2 minute. Remove from heat. Cover. Let stand 5 minutes. Pour into a buttered 8x4x2 inch mold. Chill 8 hours to season. Remove from pan and slice, mixture will be softer not firm. Dust with Tapioca flour and shape. Brown in clarified butter OR Safflower oil. Season with sea salt.

IDEAS: For additional flavor use rice cooked in Chicken Stock.
            Pour a hot vegetable puree over top when serving.
IF: Melt cheese over top of slices.

CHAPTER 2

CHICKEN FRITTERS
    1 1/2 cups all purpose flour
    3 tablespoons homemade baking powder
    3/4 teaspoon salt
    1 egg beaten
    3/4-1 cup Chicken Stock
    1 cup shredded OR chunked chicken
    1 tablespoon onion powder
    oil for frying

Whisk all dry ingredients together. Add chicken and toss. Add egg and Chicken Stock until batter becomes moistened. Drop 1 tablespoon of batter at a time into hot frying oil. Brown 3-4 minutes. Good hot. Serve plain.

IF: Dip in dark molasses, honey OR ketchup.

ROLLED CHICKEN BUNDLES
    pounded boneless chicken filets
    Celery Stuffing
    clarified butter
    oatmeal

SAUCE:
    1 cup Chicken Stock
    1 tablespoon Arrowroot
    pinch of paprika, parsley OR chives for garnish

Stuff pounded chicken filets with Celery Stuffing. Dip in clarified butter. Roll chicken in oatmeal. Bake in a preheated 350 degree oven for 25-30 minutes. Whisk Chicken Stock and Arrowroot in a sauce pan over medium high heat until broth thickens and becomes clear and slightly bubbly. Remove from heat immediately. Do not over cook. Serve over chicken. Sprinkle with paprika, parsley or fresh chives.

IF: Serve with cheese sauce over top instead of Chicken Stock.
        Substitute bread crumbs for oatmeal.

CHAPTER 2

CHICKEN LOAF
3 1/2 pounds of uncooked chicken thighs (thighs are tastier and economical)
OR 2 pounds (store bought) ground chicken
1 tablespoon onion powder
1/2 teaspoon sea salt
3 tablespoons Cream of Rice Cereal (add 1/3 cup of Chicken Stock with cereal)
OR 1/2 cooked rice
1/2 teaspoon poultry seasoning
1/2 teaspoon thyme
1/4 teaspoon paprika
3 tablespoons Safflower oil
1 egg substitute (MIX: 1/2 tablespoon Safflower oil, 1 1/2 tablespoons water and 1 tablespoon homemade baking powder)
Safflower oil OR clarified butter

Preheat oven to 375 degrees. Bone chicken thighs. Combine all food and ingredients in the food processor, except last ingredient. Chop and combine. (Do not use food processor with store bought chicken. Mix ingredients as you would meat loaf.) Oil a 10 inch loaf pan with Safflower oil and add the chicken mixture. Smooth loaf mixture on top and brush with oil. Sprinkle with parsley and paprika.

Cover loaf pan with foil. Place loaf pan into a larger pan of boiling water. Let water raise 1/2 way up sides of the loaf pan. Bake 35 minutes. Remove foil. Cook 40-45 minutes until done and no pink juices are running out of loaf when pierced. Let rest 10 minutes then slice thin.

Reserve juice from loaf and remove the fat. Use as a sauce over chicken slices thickening with Arrowroot.

BUT I CAN'T EAT THAT

CHAPTER 2

<u>CHICKEN LOAF</u> (Cont.)

GREAT SNACK: Slice Chicken Loaf thin. Fry or broil 5 minutes each side for <u>Crispy Chicken Chips</u>.

IDEAS: For richer color and flavor add spices: turmeric, curry, OR saffron threads.
Chicken Loaf is good cold on crackers OR chopped in salads.
Substitute Cream of Rye Cereal instead of rice, plus 1/2 teaspoon curry for a Far Eastern taste.
Substitute 1/2 cup Ener-G rice crispies instead of cooked rice.
Add 1/2 cup of unsweetened Applesauce before cooking loaf for a varied taste.

<u>TO GET FANCY</u>:
Wrap all <u>but</u> the bottom of a <u>cooked</u> loaf in Allergy Pie Pastry. Decorate with pie cut outs. Cook in a preheated 425 degree oven for 15 minutes until browned.

IF: Serve hot with commercial chicken gravy.
Substitute a real egg for the egg substitute. Substitute 1/2 cup mashed potatoes instead of rice.

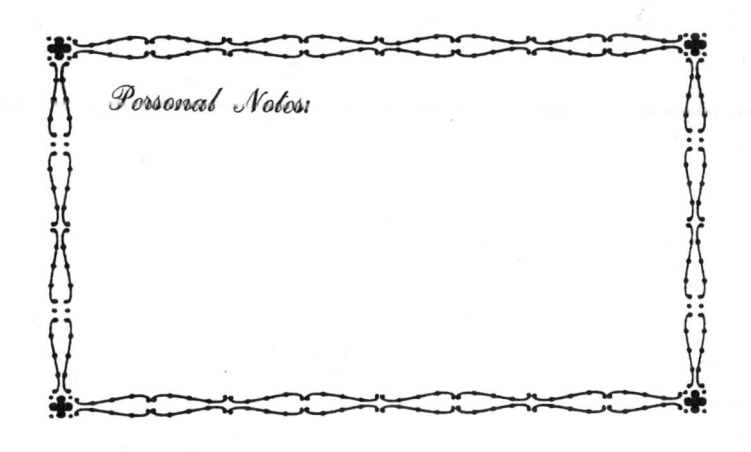

Personal Notes:

CHAPTER 2

CHICKEN ROLLS
    6 boneless chicken breasts
    3/4 cup cooked brown rice
    1 package (10 ounces) frozen chopped spinach
    1 tablespoon onion powder
    1/4 teaspoon sea salt
    1/4 teaspoon marjoram
    1/4 teaspoon crushed rosemary

Between two sheets of heavy polyurethane, pound breasts into thin fillets about 1/4 inch thick. Use the flat side of the meat mallet. Do not tear meat. Cook spinach in the microwave according to instructions. Squeeze water out by hand. (Yes, by hand. Have your children help, they'll love this job). Mix spinach with rice and remaining seasonings. (Make a paste in the food processor for 2-3 seconds if you want a smoother center.) Spread 1/3 cup of mixture over each breast. Roll chicken up, putting seam on bottom of a 12x8x2 inch glass dish. Cover and bake in a preheated 350 degree oven for 15 minutes. Uncover and bake 15 to 20 minutes more, after adding Chive Sauce.

OR: Cook chicken as above, omitting sauce for the last 20 minutes. Slice thinly and fan out on plate. Serve sauce over top. Sprinkle with paprika OR a small amount of shredded cooked carrots. With spinach inside, this makes an appealing decorative plate.

CHIVE SAUCE:
    1 cup Chicken Stock
    1 tablespoon Arrowroot
    1-2 tablespoons freshly cut chives

Whisk all ingredients together. Warm sauce slightly before adding over top of chicken. Sauce will thicken up while baking.

IF: Add 1/4 cup mozzarella cheese to spinach mix before cooking.
       Add 1 tablespoon of sour cream to spinach mix before cooking.

CHAPTER 2

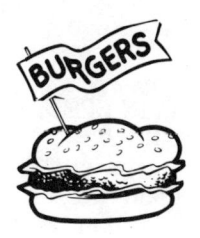

CHICKEN BURGERS
    1 pound of boneless chicken (thighs or breast)
    1/4 teaspoon poultry seasoning
    1/4 teaspoon marjoram
    1/4 teaspoon celery salt
    1 cup cooked Cream of Rice (optional)
    Rice flour

Process all ingredients in food processor for 30 seconds. Scrape to get all pieces processed 30 seconds more until mixture gets sticky and clumps. Put chicken on wax paper to make patties. Freeze uncooked. To prepare (don't thaw), take frozen patty and pat both sides with rice flour on. Fry up patties until golden brown. Eat hot or cold.

IF: Add 1/4 teaspoon sweet basil when serving patties in Allergy Spaghetti Sauce over Basic Pasta Spinach Noodles.

BUT I CAN'T EAT THAT

CHAPTER 2

CHICKEN PROTEIN SPREAD
    4 chicken thighs
    4 chicken drumsticks
    1/2 teaspoon sea salt
    1 teaspoon onion powder
    1/4 teaspoon thyme
    1/4 teaspoon poultry seasoning
    1/2 teaspoon celery salt
    optional: pinch of curry powder
    1 tablespoon parsley
    1 teaspoon sweet basil
    1/4 teaspoon paprika
    3 tablespoons to 1/4 cup Chicken Stock mixed
    with 1 tablespoon Arrowroot
    1/2-1 tablespoon chicken fat OR clarified butter

    Rinse chicken well. Cook chicken on a rack with water in bottom of pan, in a preheated 350 degree oven for 65 minutes. OR Cook chicken by boiling in a stock pot. Reduce to low and cover. Cook for 1-1 1/2 hours. Retain water for a stock base. Bone all meat while warm. Refrigerate stock and keep chicken fat that congeals on top. In the food processor puree chicken while still warm, with spices plus chicken fat butter. Whisk stock with Arrowroot and heat until thickened. Use stock to thin puree to a spreadable texture. Season with salt if needed.

IDEAS: Spread on crackers, finger sandwiches, pitas and use in making pinwheels.
            Chicken Protein Spread can be a main meal OR a nice snack.
            Chicken Protein Spread can be frozen.
            Freeze small amounts in ice cube trays.
            Chicken Spread warms up quickly in the microwave.
            Serve hot or cold.
IF: Use cream OR butter instead of chicken fat in recipe.

CHAPTER 2

CHICKEN LIVER PATE
This rich snack is wonderful, but if you have problems with mold allergies or migraines, please stay away from this.

    8 ounces fresh chicken livers
    2 tablespoons chicken fat, clarified butter OR Safflower oil
    nutmeg, salt and onion powder to taste

Wash, cut and dry chicken livers. Microwave in 1/2 cup of water, in a covered dish until done, 5 to 10 minutes on 50% power. Make sure there is no pink tissue inside. (Chicken Livers can be sautéd instead.) <u>Puree</u> livers with oils and seasonings in a food processor. Adjust seasonings as needed. Chill. Great on burritos and crackers.

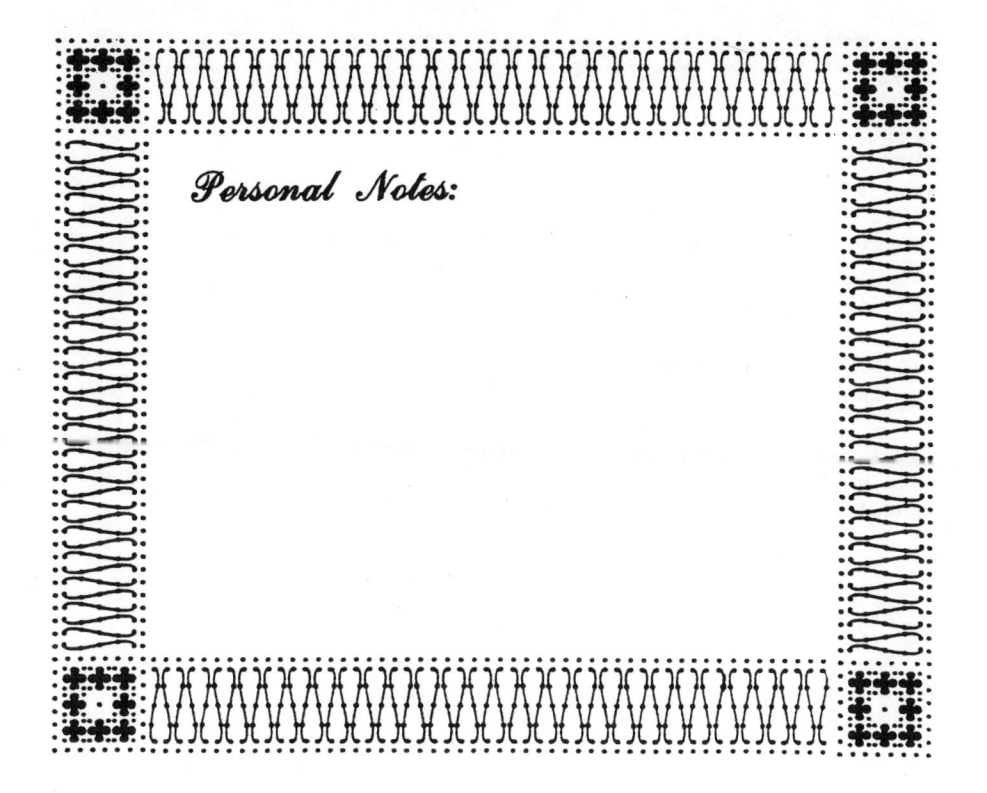

Personal Notes:

BUT I CAN'T EAT THAT

CHAPTER 2

EGGS

EGG TIMES
STOVE TOP: Try to have eggs at room temperature before cooking.
Soft boiled: Gently place eggs in the shell in boiling water for 3 minutes. Remove immediately. Crack open top, scoop out eggs and serve over toast.

Poached: Cook without shells, putting eggs directly into boiling water, cook 3 minutes, drain and serve over toast.

Hard boiled: Gently place eggs in shell into boiling water for 10-12 minutes. Remove immediately and cool in cold water. Dry and store in refrigerator until needed.

Ranch style: Crack an egg onto a buttered skillet with out breaking the yolk. Cook the fried egg until all most done then break the yolk and chop up the egg whites so the yolk spreads evenly over pieces of white when done.

Omelet: Melt clarified butter in a omelet pan or skillet. Scramble 3 eggs plus 1 tablespoon of water and cook until eggs set, over medium heat. Flip over or fold, cover until done.
*Omelets can be made with all yolks OR all whites of the eggs.

MICROWAVE: Always remove egg from shell before using in Microwave.

Soft boiled: Remove egg from shell. Place in a custard cup. Prick yolks lightly with a tooth pick, cover and cook 1-2 minutes on 50% power.

Fried: Remove egg from shell and place the on a microwavable plate. Poke yolk lightly with a tooth pick, cook covered for 1 1/2 minutes at 100% power.

Scrambled: Scramble 3 eggs plus 1 tablespoon of water and cook until eggs set, at 70% power 2-2 1/2 minutes stirring half way. Keep covered and let eggs rest for 1 minute.

Omelets: Melt clarified butter in a omelet pan or skillet. Scramble 3 eggs plus 1 tablespoon of water and cook, covered at 100% power until set for 2 minutes. Flip and cook 1 minute more at 70 % power.

BUT I CAN'T EAT THAT

CHAPTER 2

<u>IDEAL EGG USES</u> (Cont.)

Eggs make fluffier, higher volume dishes when finished, if eggs are at room temperature when using them.

Mix 1 1/2 tablespoons condensed cream of chicken soup with two eggs before cooking omelets.

Add cheese of any kind to eggs before cooking or on top of eggs after cooking.

Scrambled, fried and ranch style eggs are good in sandwiches.

Use cooked eggs, chopped in salads, Chinese foods, fried rice, burritos, sandwiches and ranch style eggs.

Fill cream puffs with scrambled eggs, top with fresh chives.

IF: Use 1 1/2 tablespoons of cream cheese in eggs omelets.

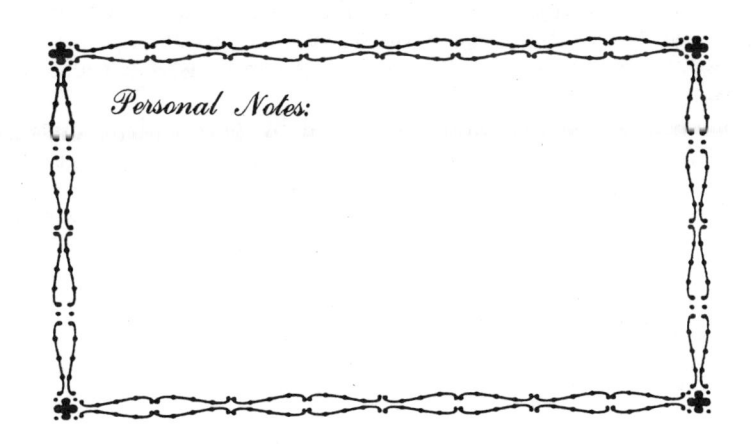

Personal Notes:

Page 53

BUT I CAN'T EAT THAT

CHAPTER 2

DUNKIN EGGS
Really fussy eaters (especially kids) think this is a fun finger food to eat. At least you can get <u>some</u> grams of protein into their bodies this way.

Soft boil 2-3 eggs (at room temperature) in boiling water for 3 minutes. Extract immediately from water. Hold hot egg with a paper napkin. Strip off the top of the egg. Scoop out the uncooked egg white out with a spoon. Pierce the yolks and pour (only the yolks) into a whiskey glass or small cup. Serve immediately with buttered toast (OR use clarified butter) sliced in long strips for dunking into the egg yolks. Salt yolks if you like.

GERMAN PANCAKES
    3 eggs at room temperature
    1/2 cup all purpose flour
    pinch of Salt Sense
    1/2 cup natural apple juice
    2 tablespoon melted clarified butter
Sauce:
    1 (8 1/4 oz.) can peaches in its own juices (no concentrates)
    1 tablespoon Arrowroot

Whisk eggs and salt until well blended. Add flour in half amounts at a time while whisking. Beat after each addition. Beat half of the juice into the batter at a time. Pour hot butter into batter while mixing. Pour the egg mixture into a hot cast iron skillet coated with butter (or lard). Bake in a preheated 400 degree oven for 15 minutes. Remove the German Pancake from the pan in one piece onto a wire rack so the bottom of the pancake does not get soggy.

Make sauce while pancake is cooking by pureeing peaches with Arrowroot in a food processor until smooth. Pour into a sauce pan and whisk constantly over medium heat until thick and slightly bubbling. Cook 7-10 minutes. Do not boil. Cut the pancake into pizza sized slices with scissors. Spread peach sauce over top. Serve hot.

IDEAS: Use other cooked or warmed fruits such as pineapple, apples or apricots. These may be chunk cut or pureed.
IF: Substitute milk instead of juice.

CHAPTER 2
GERMAN APPLE PANCAKES

3/4 cup all purpose flour
3/4 cup natural apple juice
1/4 teaspoon Salt Sense
4 eggs at room temperature
1/4 cup +3 tablespoons clarified butter
2 medium apples, sliced thin
Mix together:
2 tablespoons fructose (optional)
2 tablespoons cinnamon

Whisk eggs, juice and salt together well. Beat half of the melted butter into the mixture while hot. Use 2 tablespoons melted butter to coat two 9 inch round cake pans. Add 1/2 of the batter to each pan. Arrange apples in each pan spread out like a fan. Pour the remaining batter over top of both pans. Sprinkle with cinnamon and fructose. Cook in a preheated 400 degree oven 20-25 minutes. Serve hot.

IF: Substitute milk instead of juice.

SKILLET BREAKFAST

1 large potato
2 tablespoons Safflower oil
2 eggs
sea salt to taste
fresh chives
dash of paprika

Peel and shred one potato. Preheat a cast iron skillet on medium high heat. Add Safflower oil and heat slightly (OR use 1 tablespoon oil and 1 tablespoon butter). Add potatoes and brown both sides well. Use a splatter screen, not a lid.

Beat eggs well. Pour eggs over the top of the potatoes. Cook until eggs set, use a solid lid now. Season with sea salt, fresh chives and splash with paprika.

IDEAS: Add different chopped meats to mixture before pouring eggs in.
         Bake eggs in a 400 degree oven for 8 minutes after pouring over cooked potatoes.

IF: Melt American cheese slices over the top of the potatoes before serving.
         Substitute cooked rice spaghetti for potatoes.

Menu

Breakfast
Sweet Peach Breakfast Rice
Zucchini Bread w/Brown Rice Flour

Snack
Potato Croutons
1/2 cup of Cream of Lettuce Soup

Lunch
Just Ribs
Buttered Vegetable Pasta (Homemade)
Your Favorite Veggies w/ Curry

Snack
Jonathan's Allergy Rollups

Dinner
Meat Turnovers
Steamed Carrots
Applesauce (Homemade)
Butterflies

Snack
Allergy Lamb Loaf slices

CHAPTER 2
JONATHAN'S ALLERGY ROLLUPS

The idea for this recipe came to me from my mother. On Sunday's she always made giant pancakes that were filled with a sweet cottage cheese mixture. I remember these well because none of us were brave enough to take the first bite when she served them. The sugar and salt canister were exactly the same in her kitchen. Consequently, sometimes the filling was very salty. I finally preferred the pancakes with out the filling and just a dusting of powdered sugar. Being allergic to dairy products like my son, it worked well.

BASIC: 1 egg
          dash of sea salt
          1 cup flour
          1 cup natural style apple juice

Mix all ingredients in a blender until smooth, but do not over beat. Use batter immediately for thinner Rollups OR let it sit for 1 hour or refrigerate for 1 day, this makes the batter thicken up. Do not keep longer, mold starts after that. In large T-Fal (non stick) pan add a tad of Safflower oil OR lard (no preservatives, soy, or hydrogenated oils in it.) Pour 1/4 cup of batter into the pan and tip the pan to spread the batter very thinly, skimming with the help of the spatula. Lightly brown bottom of pancake. Flip and cook for 1 minute. Serve plain with butter and powdered sugar over the top of the Rollups. OR Fill with cooked apples, peaches, Blueberry Allergy Jam OR fresh fruit. Roll and serve hot. With breakfast stuffings, recipe makes 7-8 Rollups. Reheat frozen Rollups with butter in the microwave for 30 seconds on high setting. Nice with a dusting of powdered sugar and or fresh lemon juice and butter OR whatever your favorite topping is.

IDEAS: Can add 1/2 teaspoon cinnamon, 3/4 tablespoon carob
          OR 1 tablespoon fructose
          Use other flours: rye, oat, rice, etc.
IF: Filing-Pinch of salt
          1 cup dry ricotta
          1 egg yolk
          2 tablespoons fructose
          1/2 teaspoon cinnamon

Fill and bake in a preheated 350 degree oven for 15 minutes adding butter over the top for moisture.
For <u>DESSERT ROLLUPS</u>: Add 2-3 tablespoons of Carob, plus 2 tablespoons of fructose plus 1/2 teaspoon cinnamon.
IF: Substitute: milk for juice; butter for oil; add 2-3
          more tablespoons of Carob.

CHAPTER 2

FISH

NO TURN BASIC FISH FORMULAS

BAKED
Put 1 1/2 pounds of cleaned fish fillets oiled with Safflower oil in a single layer on an oiled baking sheet. Bake in a preheated 400 degree oven for 15-20 minutes. Thicken fish juices with Arrowroot and sprinkle with parsley.

BROILED
Put 1 1/2 pounds of cleaned fish fillets oiled with Safflower oil in a single layer on an oiled baking sheet with a lip. Add a small amount of water, but do not cover fish with water. Broil 12 minutes. Do not turn fish over.

IF: Put a thick covering of mayo over top of fish. Sprinkle with bread crumbs. Dot with butter. Sprinkle with paprika and cook.

BAKED AND STUFFED
Put Celery Stuffing between 2 fish fillets. Oil top and bottom of fish with Safflower oil. Sprinkle top with Fish Seasonings. Bake on a greased pan in a preheated 400 degree oven for 25-35 minutes. If fish flakes it's done.

STEAMED
In a steamer, bring water to a boil. Place fish on a steamer rack so no water is touching the fish. Cover and steam. Thin fish filets cook in 5 minutes, steaks cook in 7 minutes or until fish flakes easily with a fork. Steam vegetables around the fish. OR add the fish to the veggies during the last 5 minutes if the veggies need a longer steam bath.

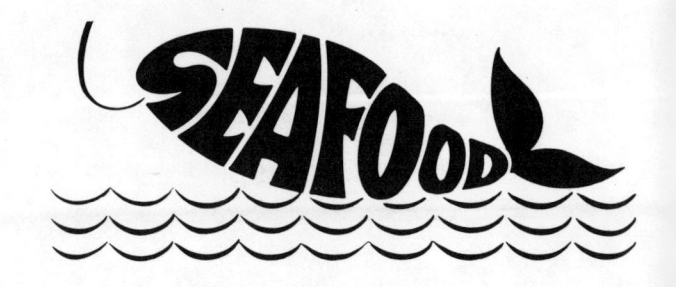

BUT I CAN'T EAT THAT

CHAPTER 2

<u>FISH</u> (Cont.)

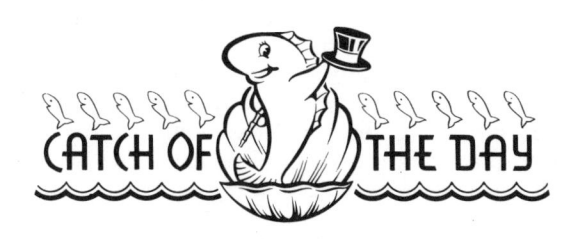

CATCH OF THE DAY

STEAK
Examples to use for cooking fish steaks are Swordfish and Halibut that are 1/2 inch thick. Rinse fish and dry with paper towels. Score underside of fish so it will not curl up when cooking. Oil both sides with Safflower oil and season with sea salt on the top and the bottom. Add a small amount of liquid to the bottom of the pan. Cook on the top rack 4 inches from the broiler coils. Cook 6 minutes. Fish will flake with a fork when done. Do not turn. Can use clarified butter instead of oil.

PAN FRIED
In a hot skillet heat enough Safflower oil to cover the bottom of a pan. You can dust fish with Tapioca flour first. Add fish fillets to hot oil. Cook until browned. Turn and cook other side until brown.

SAUCE
Using leftover pan juices from fish recipe makes a delicious "gravy" thickened with Arrowroot. However, the sauce is almost colorless, therefore very unappetizing. Adding paprika, turmeric or dill herbs will give the dish eye appeal, aroma and flavor. Serve over hot fish.

CHAPTER 2
SEAFOOD PILAF
    1 tablespoon onion powder
    1 tablespoon Safflower oil
    1 package rice pilaf (OR homemade mixture)
    1 pound package of fish (cut into 1 inch cubes)
    1 pound of green beans (cooked)

In a skillet, sauté fish until done. Chop green beans smaller and mix in fish. Mix rice and spices together. Sauté until hot and rice is browned. Serve with parsley sprigs and paprika.

FISH AND SPINACH WRAPS
    1 pound of fresh spinach OR 1, 10 oz. box of frozen spinach
    6-7 fillets of Sole
    1/2 teaspoon Fish Spices
    dash of nutmeg
    1/2 tablespoon onion powder
    Safflower oil OR clarified butter
    paprika

Clean and cook spinach. Chop. (If using frozen spinach, squeeze all water out after cooking.) Sauté spinach in oil with nutmeg and onion powder. Spread one layer of spinach on one side of each fish fillet. Brush an 8 inch round cake pan with oil. Roll up fillet with spinach. Place fish on it's side and stack side by side to fit in pan. (Like cinnamon rolls are placed.) Brush the tops of the fish with oil. Sprinkle with paprika. Cover pan with tin foil. Bake in a preheated 400 degree oven for 25-35 minutes.

TUNA PATTIES
    6 ounces drained tuna (in water)
    1 tablespoon Safflower oil
    1/4 cup finely chopped celery
    onion powder to taste
    1 egg (OR-1 1/2 tablespoons Safflower oil with 1 1/2 tablespoons water and 1 teaspoon homemade baking powder)
    Tapioca flour

Mince tuna in the food processor. Mix all ingredients together. Shape into patties. Pat flour or bread crumbs on both sides of patty. Heat Safflower oil in skillet until hot. Fry up patties until brown and crispy on both sides. Serve hot or cold.
IF: Substitute homemade bread crumbs for Tapioca flour.

CHAPTER 2

LAMB, PORK, AND VEAL

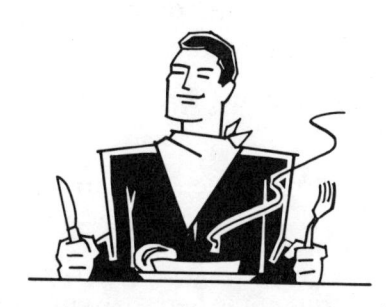

LAMB ROAST using-
LEG OF LAMB
Lamb should be well cooked. A 6 to 6 1/2 pound leg of lamb feeds 4 to 5 people. Place fat side up for roasting. Insert meat thermometer in thickest section to read 180 degrees when cooked. Roast 325-350 degrees for 30-35 minutes per pound. Serve hot.

LAMB CHOPS
Broil lamb chops for 5 minutes or until blood rises to top. Turn lamb chops over and broil other side 3 minutes more.

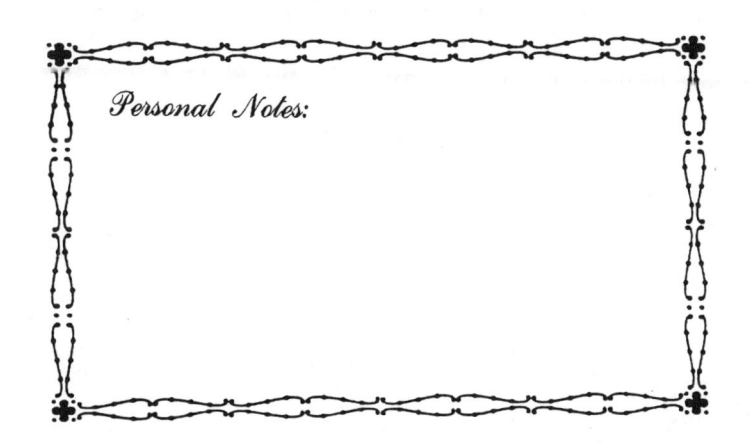

Personal Notes:

CHAPTER 2

LAMB POT PIE
- 3 cups cooked lamb
- One 5 ounce package frozen pea pods
- 3/4 cup diced cooked carrots
- 1-1 1/2 cups Lamb Stock
- 1 pastry top with lamb cutouts for decorations
- 1/2 teaspoon marjoram
- 1 teaspoon thyme
- 1 1/2-2 tablespoons Tapioca flour OR Arrowroot

Whisk Tapioca flour or Arrowroot into cold Lamb Stock. Add lamb and vegetables together. Place into a glass pie pan. Cover with pastry top, pinch edges tight. For decoration paste pastry cut outs on top with water. Prick top before cooking for steam to escape. Bake in a preheated 350 degree oven for 45 minutes or until bubbly.

PASTRY TOP (Makes two tops)
- 2 cups all purpose flour
- 1 teaspoon homemade baking powder
- 1 teaspoon Salt Sense
- 1/2 cup lard (no preservatives)
- 1/2 cup cold water (plus 1 tablespoon more if too dry)

With a wire whisk blend flour, salt and baking powder well. Cut in lard with pastry cutter (OR two knives) until mixture looks like the size of small peas. With a fork gently mix in water, to make a dough. Do not overwork. Cut dough in half. Roll dough out between two sheets of wax paper. Freezes extra top.

IDEAS: For quicker cooking time:
Precook pastry top on parchment paper on a cookie sheet in preheated 425 degrees for 8-10 minutes until browned.
Thicken cold stock with Arrowroot over medium high heat, stirring constantly. While stock is hot, add precooked pastry top to cover and serve.

IF: Can add diced potatoes to body of pie.
Brush with a egg white wash over pastry for quicker browning.

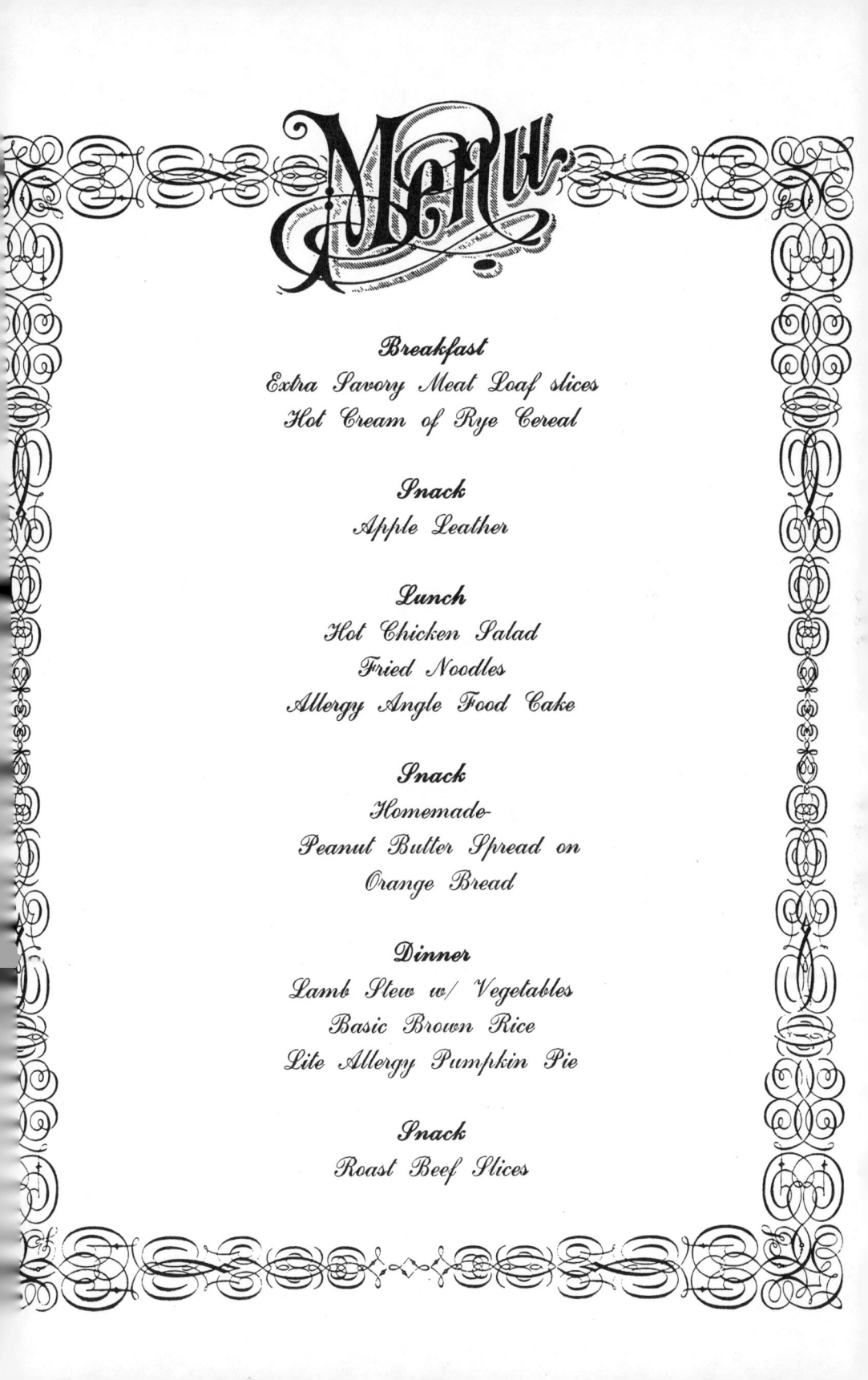

Menu

Breakfast
Extra Savory Meat Loaf slices
Hot Cream of Rye Cereal

Snack
Apple Leather

Lunch
Hot Chicken Salad
Fried Noodles
Allergy Angle Food Cake

Snack
Homemade
Peanut Butter Spread on
Orange Bread

Dinner
Lamb Stew w/ Vegetables
Basic Brown Rice
Lite Allergy Pumpkin Pie

Snack
Roast Beef Slices

CHAPTER 2

LAMB STEW

1 1/2 pounds cubed lamb
1 tablespoon onion powder
2 cups Lamb Stock
lard for browning
1 teaspoon sweet basil
dash of oregano
1/3 cup Tapioca flour
2 tablespoons parsley
2 celery stalks (cut chunky)
2 carrots (cut chunky)
1/2 teaspoon sea salt
Lard for browning

Place all spices into a plastic bag with the flour. Place lamb chunks in bag and shake until coated. Brown the lamb in a preheated heavy iron skillet with lard. Sauté vegetables 5 minutes in lamb juices left in the skillet. Remove all foods from the pan. Add lamb broth scraping the tidbits from the bottom of the pan. Bring to a boil. Add the meat and vegetables. Cover skillet with foil. Cook on low for 1 hour. OR put stew in a Crock Pot and cook on low for 10-12 hours. Add extra Tapioca flour to thicken sauce, 1/2 hour before the stew is finished cooking. Serve over rice OR Basic Tomato Pasta.

IF: Add 2 cups stewed tomatoes, garlic powder and 1 tablespoon of lemon juice for a sharper flavor.
Serve with baked potatoes.

CHAPTER 2

LAMB WRAP
    1 pound ground lamb
    Allergy Pie Crust, bread dough, OR phyllo brushed with clarified butter
    1 package (10 ounces) chopped spinach
    1 tablespoon onion powder
    1/4 teaspoon curry powder
    1/4 teaspoon sea salt
    1/2 cups cooked rice
    1 Egg Substitute: Mix together: 1/2 tablespoon oil, 1 1/2 tablespoon water, 1 teaspoon homemade baking powder

Sauté ground lamb until just done in a T-Fal pan with no added oils. Drain juices after cooking and discard. Add all spices to the lamb. While mixing spices in, break up any large lumps of lamb. Microwave spinach in package per instructions on box. Squeeze out all moisture in the spinach with your hands (its the only way!) Mix spinach with lamb mixture forming it into a loaf. Cover loaf with a thin layer of Allergy Pie Crust. Place seam side down on bottom of pan. Brush with clarified butter. Cook in a preheated 375 degree oven for 30 minutes. Loaf should be nicely browned when finished.

IF: Replace egg substitute of oil, water, and baking soda with 1-2 real eggs.
      Add 1/2 cup sour cream to lamb mixture before making it into a loaf.
      Add 1/2 cup grated cheese to lamb mixture before making it into a loaf.
      Brush pastry with 1 egg white and 1 teaspoon water.

CHAPTER 2

ALLERGY LAMB LOAF
1 1/2 pounds ground lamb
3 tablespoons Cream of Brown Rice Cereal
1/3 cup water
1/2 cup finely chopped celery (sauté)
3 tablespoons dried parsley
1 tablespoon onion powder
1/4 teaspoon thyme, marjoram, celery salt and curry
1/2 teaspoon sea salt
1 Egg Substitute (1 1/2 tablespoon Safflower oil, 1 1/2 tablespoon water mixed with 1 teaspoon homemade baking powder)
paprika

Mix all ingredients, except paprika, by hand using a light touch. Line a 3x1x4 inch bread tin with wax paper. Put meat into mold, pressing lightly with your hands or the back of a spoon. Turn out onto a rack and remove the wax paper. Sprinkle the top with paprika. Bake in a preheated 350 degree oven for about 1 hour. Check to see that no pink juices are run out of loaf when pierced. If so, bake 10 more minutes. Loaf should be browned when finished.

IDEAS: Add 1-2 cups grated cooked carrots OR cauliflower (sautéd) to mixture before cooking.
Serve hot or cold.
Slice and freeze for lunches. Loaf can be frozen and reheated in the microwave. Defrost 1-3 slices on 30 percent power for 1 1/2 minutes. Reheat on 80 percent power about 30 seconds per side.
Allergy Lamb Loaf mixture is great cooked as burgers.

IF: Use evaporated milk OR tomato sauce instead of 1/3 cup water.
After loaf is cooked melt slices of Muenster, brick or mozzarella cheese over top before serving.
You can use a real egg instead of the egg substitute.

BUT I CAN'T EAT THAT

CHAPTER 2

<u>LAMB MEATBALLS IN WHITE SAUCE</u>
Using the recipe for Allergy Lamb Loaf, make 1-2 inch meatballs with the mixture. Place on a wire rack. Bake in a preheated 400 degree oven for 20 minutes.

<u>WHITE SAUCE</u>
        1 cup Lamb Stock
        1/2 teaspoon dill weed
        1 tablespoon Arrowroot

Combine all ingredients. Whisk sauce over medium heat until thick. Add hot meatballs to White Sauce. Serve over hot brown rice. Sprinkle fresh parsley adding a tad of paprika over the top for garnish.

IDEAS: Serve over homemade Pasta.
             You can add a small amount of your favorite vegetables to the white sauce for color.

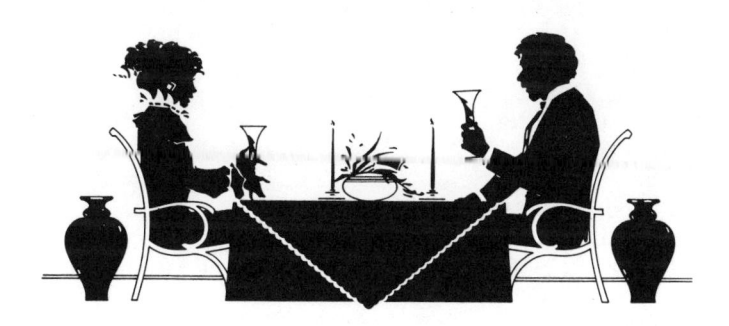

BUT I CAN'T EAT THAT

CHAPTER 2

PORK

BASIC PORK CHOPS

BAKED
Rinse and dry pork chops before cooking. Season with sea salt or other spices. Place on a pan with a rack allowing fat to drip off while cooking. Place a tad of clarified butter OR lard (no preservatives) on top for extra flavor. Bake in a preheated 350 degree oven for 45 minutes or until browned; 1 hour for very thick pork chops.

BRAISED
In an iron skillet, preheat lard (no preservatives) on medium high heat. Brown both sides of chops. Add 1 cup Chicken Stock to pan and bring to a boil. Cover tightly with a lid or aluminum foil. Turn heat down to low. Simmer for 30 minutes. Drain liquid to make sauce. Dissolve 1 tablespoon Arrowroot in 2 tablespoons cold water. Slowly add to stock as a thickener for sauce. Heat on medium, stirring constantly until sauce thickens. Do not boil. Adjust seasonings. Add pork chops and serve.

GRILLED
It's safer for people with allergies not to use gas grills and starter fluids. When using charcoal briquettes an electric starter is best.
    Boil pork chops in water for 5-10 minutes to ensure cooking all the way through and to remove excess fat that will cause the fire to flame. Put pork chops directly over coals on grill. Cook 7-10 minutes per side. Cut for color check, if color is pink, cook 5 minutes more on each side. Grilled chops cook best when using thinner pork chops. Thicker chops must be turned more frequently and cooked 10-15 minutes longer.

PORK TENDERLOIN
Pork Tenderloin is a delightful piece of meat with no bones. Simply slice it up and sauté. Use raw pork tenderloin for shishkebabs, Chinese dishes. Use cooked tenderloins minced in omelets, salads, burittos OR stuffed in pita pockets.
    You can bake the tenderloin whole as a roast. Brush with Seasoned Butter OR Safflower oil. Bake in a preheated 350 degree oven for 1 hour. Test to see if roast is done by cutting, if the juices that run out of a cut are pink, the roast needs to be cooked for 10 minutes more.

BUT I CAN'T EAT THAT

CHAPTER 2

PORK ROAST
Always cook pork roast thoroughly. Rub meat with paprika, Safflower oil, onion powder and Tapioca flour. A 4 to 6 pound pork roast will serve 4 people. Preheat oven to 350 degrees. Cook 2 hours for a 4 pound roast, 3 hours for a 6 pound roast.

A plain roast (not seasoned) makes its own crispy crust when the fat on top of the roast cooks. Do not trim the fat (use this to your advantage for automatic basting). It is best to use a meat thermometer to ensure perfection. When the roast is done, the inside temperature should register 185 degrees. No pink juices should run out of a puncture when the roast is finished cooking.

Add water to the bottom of the pan to make Au juice. Refrigerate liquid (if possible) to remove fats that harden on the surface. Add Arrowroot or Tapioca flour to thicken. Serve hot. Great when sliced cold for snacking OR cubed for salads, pitas OR burritos.

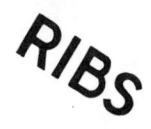

RIBS

JUST RIBS (WESTERN SPARE RIBS)

Boil ribs in salted hot water for 10 minutes. Drain. Place on a T-Fal cookie sheet OR on a slotted rack. Cook 45 minutes in a 350 degree preheated oven. If you do not boil first, then cook 1 hour or longer. If ribs are super thick, 2 inches or larger, turn over half way through cooking time. If using a T-Fal sheet, drain greases at this time. The ribs cooked flat on the T-Fal will have a browned, crisper crust. The ribs cooked on the slotted rack are not so crusty, but are just as good. Season with sea salt and dig in. Allow 3 ribs per big appetite.

BUT I CAN'T EAT THAT

CHAPTER 2

<u>SWEET PORK CUTLETS</u>
    1 pound pork cutlets
    1 teaspoon Arrowroot
    1/4 teaspoon thyme
    1/4 teaspoon onion powder
    2 tablespoons Safflower oil and 1 tablespoon clarified butter
    1/2 cup natural apple juice

    Pound cutlets thin between 2 sheets of thick polyurethane with <u>flat</u> side of meat tenderizing hammer. Do not tear meat. Season with spices. Mix oil and butter in an iron skillet over medium high heat. Sauté cutlets until cooked through (3 minutes each side). Remove and keep warm. Pour fat out of pan. Whisk apple juice and Arrowroot together adding to the hot pan, scraping any residue from the pan into the sauce. When the sauce thickens, pour over cutlets and serve hot.

IDEAS: Microwave using a browning dish and serve cutlets plain.
IF: Use 1/4 cup brandy instead of apple juice and reduce.
          Use an apple juice concentrate for a sweeter taste.

<u>ALLERGY SAUSAGE PATTIES</u>

<u>Small</u>	<u>Large</u>	<u>Ingredients</u>
1 pound	2 pounds	ground pork
1/4 tsp.	1/2 tsp.	thyme
1/4 tsp.	1/2 tsp.	marjoram
1/4 tsp.	1/2 tsp.	sweet basil
3/4 tsp.	1 1/2 tsp	Salt Sense
1/3 cup	2/3 cup	water
		Safflower Oil

    Mix all ingredients together thoroughly, for a smaller batch OR a larger batch. Shape into thinner (4 inch diameter) patties. Fry in Safflower oil until brown on both sides. Make sure patties are <u>thoroughly</u> cooked. Extra time will not hurt these babies. Sausage patties can be kept warm for a long time without becoming tough. Freeze with or without cooking patties.

IDEAS: Use all pork, all beef OR 1/2 pork and 1/2 beef mixture.
          (Your preference.)
IF: Adding 2 teaspoons of sage is nice.
          To make spicier patties add a good dash of pepper.

CHAPTER 2

PORK POT PIE WITH VEGETABLES
    3 cups cooked pork
    1 (10 ounce) package frozen combo of carrots, cauliflower, and green beans
    1 to 1 1/2 cups Chicken Stock
    1/2 teaspoon marjoram
    1 pastry top with pig cutouts for decorations
    1 1/2-2 tablespoons Tapioca flour

Combine 1 1/2 to 2 tablespoons (For Arrowroot-see note below) Tapioca flour to Chicken Stock when its cold. Mix in pork and vegetables. Cover with pastry top, pinch edges tight. Prick top to let steam escape. Brush backs of cutouts with water and stick to top of pie. Bake in a preheated 350 degree oven for 45 minutes until bubbly.

Note: If using Arrowroot do not let pie boil. Or heat all in a pan and just brown Pastry Top for 10 minutes in a 450 degree oven on a cookie sheet.

PASTRY TOP (Makes two tops)
    2 cups all purpose flour
    1 teaspoon homemade baking powder
    1 teaspoon Salt Sense
    1/4 cup butter and 1/4 cup lard (no preservatives)
    1/2 cup cold water and 1 tablespoon (if too dry)

With a wire whisk blend flour, salt and baking powder well. Cut in lard with pastry cutter (OR two knives) until mixture resembles the size of small peas. With fork gently mix water to make a dough. Do not overwork. If too dry add 1 tablespoon of water at a time as needed. Divide dough in half. Roll out between two sheets of wax paper. Freeze extra top.

IDEAS: For quicker cooking time:
            Precook pastry top on parchment paper on cookie sheet at preheated 425 degrees for 8-10 minutes until browned. Thicken cold broth with Arrowroot over medium high heat, stirring constantly. Stock will become thick. Add precooked pastry top to cover and serve.

IF: Can add corn and potatoes to Chicken Stock.
            Brush with egg white wash over pastry for quicker browning.

BUT I CAN'T EAT THAT

CHAPTER 2

PORK CITY CHICKEN
    3 pounds pork chops
    1/2 cup Tapioca flour
    1/4 teaspoon each sweet basil, celery salt,
    sea salt, onion powder and thyme
    3 tablespoons lard (no preservative)
    1 1/2 cup Chicken Stock
    1-2 tablespoons Arrowroot
    2 tablespoons of cold water

    Cut pork into 1 to 1 1/2 inch square pieces. Skewer pork pieces onto wood sticks. In a plastic bag add Tapioca flour and your favorite seasonings OR 1/4 teaspoon basil, celery salt, sea salt, onion powder, paprika and thyme. Drop city chicken pieces on sticks, into bag one at a time. Close bag and shake to coat. Set aside. In a heavy cast iron skillet, heat lard on medium high heat. Brown all sides of city chicken. Discard any leftover lard in pan. If any Tapioca flour is left, whisk it into Chicken Stock adding to skillet with meat. Bring liquid to a boil. Cover with aluminum foil, reduce to low and simmer. Simmer 45 minutes to 1 hour. Remove meat when done and keep warm with foil. If juices are not thick enough for gravy, add Arrowroot blending with cold water then add to sauce. Whisk constantly over medium heat until thick. Add seasonings, sea salt and meat to gravy, then serve.

CHAPTER 2

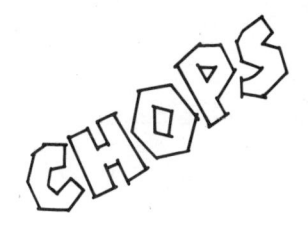

CHOPS

PORK CHOP SKILLET DINNER

  4 thick pork chops
  1/2 cup uncooked brown rice
  2-3 tablespoons lard OR Safflower oil
  1 tablespoon onion powder
  2-3 tablespoons chopped celery
  1/4 teaspoon each marjoram, thyme and sea salt
  1 cup Chicken Stock

In large cast iron skillet heat oil on medium high heat. Brown pork chops on both sides then remove from skillet. In the meat juices and oils on bottom of pan sauté rice, celery, and spices for 5 minutes. Add stock, bring to boil. Remove pan from the heat. Add rice to the skillet and place pork chops on top. Tightly cover with aluminum foil. Cook in preheated 350 degree oven for 1 hour.

IDEAS: Add cut vegetables on top of the pork chops before putting into the oven and cook your whole supper in one pan. Hardly any clean-up!

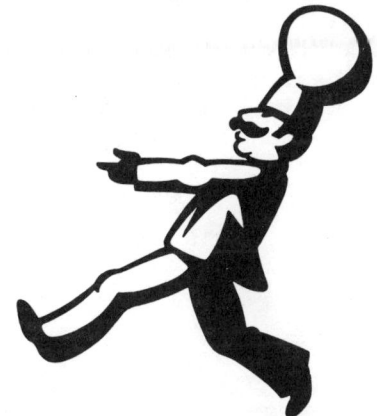

BUT I CAN'T EAT THAT

CHAPTER 2

VEAL

Ground veal is a good meat to use in combination with other meats, such as in meatloaf. (See Allergy Meatloaf and Pureed Meat) Many people do not realize how tasty it is by itself. When you are limited in food selection veal is a welcome change.

VEAL PATTIES (PLAIN)
1 pound ground veal

Shape into 4 thick patties. Preheat a cast iron skillet with a small amount of lard OR Safflower oil. Sprinkle sea salt on bottom of pan. Add patty, covering the pan with a splash guard, do not use a solid lid. When blood comes to top of the patty it is time to turn the patty over. When same thing occurs to this side your veal patty is done to perfection. Total cooking time is 10-12 minutes.

VEAL PATTIES (SPICED)
1 pound ground veal
1/4 cup parsley
1/4 teaspoon sea salt
1/4 teaspoon thyme
1/4 teaspoon sweet basil
1/8 teaspoon paprika
1/8 teaspoon nutmeg

Mix veal with all spices. Put meat in a covered bowl and leave over night in the refrigerator. In the morning, press veal into thinner patties that cook quickly. Brown both sides in Safflower oil in a preheated skillet. Serve hot. Great for breakfast patties.

IF: Add 1/4 teaspoon sage to mixture.

CHAPTER 2

<u>VEAL SCALLOPINI CACCIATORE</u>
    2 pounds scalloped veal
    1/2 cup Tapioca flour
    1/2 teaspoon sea salt
    clarified butter or Safflower oil (or half butter and half oil)
    4-5 cups Allergy Spaghetti Sauce

Dust veal with flour and salt. Heat sauce in microwave 4-5 minutes on 100% power. Sauté veal in oils and mix with hot sauce. Put veal and sauce in a casserole and cover. Bake in a preheated 400 degree oven for 20-25 minutes. Garnish with parsley.

IDEAS: When using tougher cuts such as leg or shoulder, cook in crock pot for 8-10 hours on low.
IF: Add 8 ounces shredded mozzarella cheese to top of casserole before cooking in the oven.

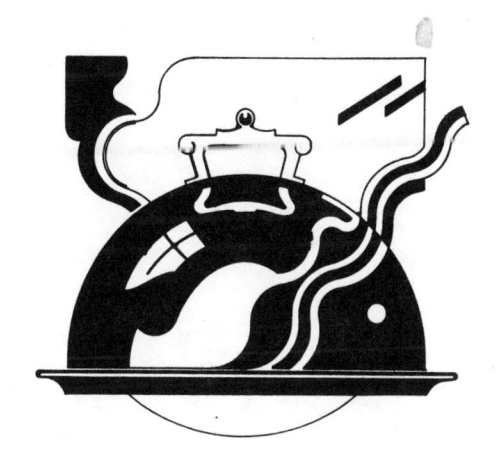

BUT I CAN'T EAT THAT

CHAPTER 2

TURKEY

TURKEY HASH
    1-2 tablespoons onion powder
    1 cup chopped celery OR 1 teaspoon celery salt
    2 tablespoons clarified butter + 2 tablespoons Safflower oil
    2 cups diced cooked turkey
    2 cups diced cooked potatoes
    1/2 cup Chicken Stock
    1/2 teaspoon tarragon
    1/2 teaspoon poultry seasoning
    1/2 teaspoon sea salt
    Safflower oil

Sauté potatoes in oil until well browned. Add turkey and remaining ingredients to skillet. Bring stock to a boil, reduce heat to low and simmer. Simmer 15 minutes until liquid reduces and evaporates.

IDEAS: Exchange brown rice OR long grain white rice for potatoes. Sauté rice until it's crispy on medium high heat.
You can add 1/2 cup vegetables of your choice, sweet peas, green beans, carrots, etc.

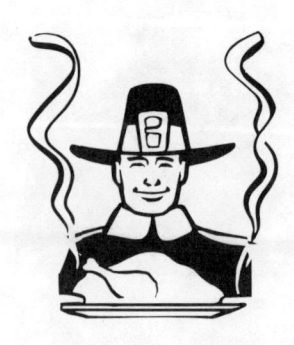

CHAPTER 2

GROUND TURKEY

Fresh ground turkey is sold in every supermarket. Check the ingredients on the label for additives and preservatives. Ground turkey can be substituted in many recipes that require a ground meat OR poultry. Here is a good Chinese turkey meatball recipe to try out on your taste buds.

C/T MEATBALLS
   1 pound ground turkey
   3 tablespoons Cream of Brown Rice Cereal
   1/3 cup water
   1/4 teaspoon sea salt
   1/4 teaspoon poultry seasoning
   Safflower oil for cooking
   1 cup Chicken Stock
   2 ribs Bok Choy
   4 carrots
   5-6 leaves of Napa cabbage
   1 tablespoons Tapioca flour

Mix first five ingredients together and form meatballs, 1 inch round. Brown meatballs in hot oil, using medium high heat. Cut and slice vegetables. In a sauce pan, bring Chicken Stock to a boil and add veggies. Cook for 10 minutes or until veggies are done. (Using precooked veggies speeds up this process.) Remove veggies with a slotted spoon and keep warm. Whisk Tapioca flour and 1 tablespoon of cold water (OR stock), then add to boiling stock stirring until it thickens. Add vegetables and meatballs to stock. Cover and cook 5 minutes more. Mixture should be thick and bubbly. Serve over brown rice, rice noodles OR serve plain.

CHAPTER 2

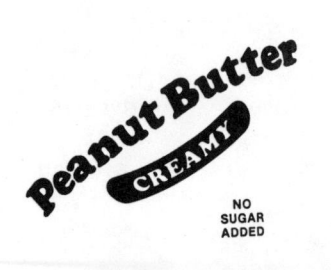

MISCELLANEOUS

HOMEMADE PEANUT BUTTER

12 ounces unsalted dry roasted peanuts
1-2 tablespoons Safflower oil

Using food processor, add peanuts and process until dry and pasty (3-5 minutes). Slowly add 1 tablespoon of oil to thin and moisten peanut butter. If needed very carefully add one more tablespoon of oil. Test often by turning motor off and poking mixture with your finger. (Hint: If in doubt, do not add extra oil.) Keep refrigerated.

IDEAS: If you like a sweeter peanut butter add up to 3 tablespoons of fructose or molasses.
If you like chunky peanut butter, add 1/2 cup nuts at the end to slightly chop them into the mixture.

IF: If you like a sweeter peanut butter add up to 3 tablespoons of cane sugar.

HOMEMADE PEANUT BUTTER SPREAD

1/2 cup natural peanut butter (no sugar)
1/2 cup natural applesauce (no sugar)
1/4 cup raisins

Puree all ingredients in the food processor just until blended. Spread on top of Heavy English Muffin Bread for breakfast or a snack any time. Keep remaining spread refrigerated.

IF: Sesame seeds OR carob chips can be added for fun.

BUT I CAN'T EAT THAT

CHAPTER 2

<u>MEAT TURNOVERS</u>
Dough:
    1 package dry yeast
    1 cup warm water (110 degrees)
    1 tablespoon sugar OR fructose
    (1 tablespoon Safflower oil for bowl)
    1/2 teaspoon Salt Sense
    1-2 1/2 cups all purpose flour

    Dissolve yeast in warm water with sugar. Add remaining ingredients to flour. Mix in yeast. Knead for 5 minutes. Turn into a greased bowl using 1 tablespoon Safflower oil. Raise 1 hour or until dough doubles. Punch down and divide into 10 parts. Roll each part into 5 inch circles. Fill with 3 tablespoons of filling. Fold over and pinch close. Dip a fork into water and flute edges closed. Cover turnovers with a damp linen towel and let raise until double, 1 hour. Bake in a preheated 375 degree oven for 20-25 minutes. Turnovers should be light brown.

<u>MEAT MIXTURE</u>: (beef, lamb, veal, turkey or chicken)
    Use Meatloaf Recipes for separate meats. Brown the ground meat. Mix in 1 egg and spices. Puree meat in the food processor. You can fill turnovers with a chunkier cut meat OR use diced meat from a roast.

IDEAS:	All vegetable turnovers can be made using <u>pre-cooked</u> vegetables.
	Use a pasta machine to roll out the dough smoother and thinner.
IF:	Any cheeses can be added to turnovers before folding flap closed.

CHAPTER 2

HEIDI'S NO CHEESE RAVIOLI
1 recipe of Basic: Pasta-Ravioli (Dough)
(Recipe includes dough size)

MEAT FILLING:
    1, 3 ounce hamburger patty (ground sirloin)
    1, 3 ounce veal patty
    1 Egg Substitute (1 1/2 tablespoon Safflower oil, 1 1/2 tablespoon water, 1 teaspoon homemade baking powder)
    paprika, onion powder and sea salt to taste

Combine meats and cook until just done. In food processor combine cooked meats with egg substitute. Add 2-3 shakes of paprika, onion powder and sea salt to mixture and continue processing until meat turns into a paste. With a small watermelon scooper place 1 teaspoon of meat mixture on Ravioli dough across in even rows. Mist lightly with water from a spray bottle over top of dough with the meat on it. Place the top dough over meatballs and press the air out. Use a small wooden rod to roll in between the meat piles. Cut and pinch edges closed with a fork. Cook in boiling water (with or without salt) 15-20 minutes until dough is soft. Drain and add to hot Allergy Spaghetti Sauce. Makes 12-16 squares.

IDEAS: Use the extra dough as noodles, slice thinly and freeze.
              Freeze separately on a cookie sheet (for 1 hour in the freezer) then package in one bag.
IF: Add Parmesan or Romano cheese to meat mixture.
              You can use real grated onions or garlic in meat mixture.
              You can use a real egg instead of the Egg Substitute.

Chapter 3

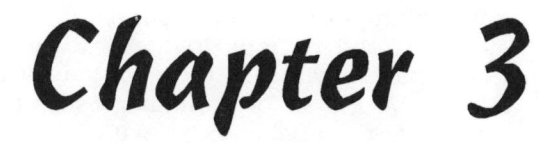

Carbohydrates

BUT I CAN'T EAT THAT

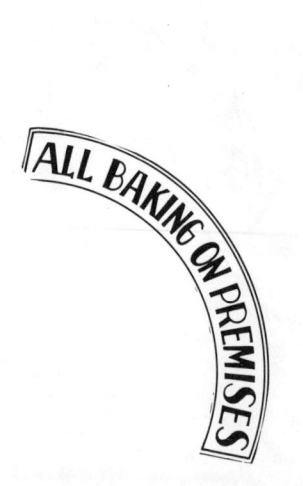

CHAPTER 3

ALL BAKING ON PREMISES

BREADS

If you are not into baking bread, Italian specialty shops have two breads with no preservatives and no milk in them. By name they are Ciabatta and Sopette. The bakery will slice them for you. If the bread is not eaten that day it must be frozen for without preservatives the loaf stales in one day. (These loaves are baked fresh daily.) Before freezing, I suggest inserting wax paper in between the slices for easier removal when individual pieces are wanted. Also a double wrap outside the loaf provides more protection from freezer burn and ice build up, which makes the bread soggy when reheating. This way you have fresh bread any time.

Cooking breads without yeast and substituting different flours has not been too successful and the loaves were not tasty. Here's where the Ener-G-Co. (address in Safe and Accessible Foods) produces a decent loaf worth trying. It's called their Brown Rice Bread, yeast free.

CORN BREAD seems to be a tough one to duplicate without milk or buttermilk. Pepperidge Farms does carry a frozen corn muffin that I nuke in the microwave and then brown the top in the oven. This works for our allergies so you might want to check it out for yours. (They are lower in milk products and sugar and they do taste great.)

CHAPTER 3

BASIC: FRENCH BREAD

Large	Small	Ingredients
1 1/2	1	packet dry active yeast
1	1 3/4	cups warm water (110 degrees)
3 1/4	5-5 1/2	cups all purpose flour OR bread flour
1	1/2	teaspoon sea salt

Proof yeast by adding warm water to sugar and letting it stand covered until foamy, 5-10 minutes. Slowly mix in flour by hand forming a stiff dough. Knead on a floured board 8-10 minutes until no longer sticky. OR in a food processor blend the dry ingredients (all but 1/2 cup flour) for 5 seconds. With the motor running add yeast until mixture forms a ball around the blade. Add 1 tablespoon of flour at a time if dough is too moist. Run motor 20 seconds. Process another 40 seconds to knead. Turn dough out into a greased bowl. Cover and let rise in a draft free, warm area 1-1 1/2 hours until doubled in bulk. If too cold, place dough in a cold electric oven with a pan of boiling water underneath the bowl. (This method is terrific!)

Punch dough down and divide in half for 2 loaves OR in fourths for mini-loaves OR rolls. Let dough rise 1 hour again. Preheat oven 425 degrees. Boil water in a teakettle to have ready. Glaze with 1 teaspoon corn starch mixed with 1/2 cup water [IF: 1 egg white mixed with 1 tablespoon cold water]. Slash with a razor blade in three traditional diagonal lines on tops of loaves/rolls. Place a narrow pan of hot water on bottom rack. Bake 25-35 minutes for loaves, 14-15 minutes for rolls. Brush glaze again on top 1/2 way through cooking. The bread should sound hollow when tapped on the bottom. For softer crusts, spray a water mist loafs several times while cooking

CUT BISCUITS-with Basic French Bread
Follow above recipe and roll out dough after first raising. Roll 1/2 inch thick. Cut biscuits out with a sharp press. Place on a non greased T-Fal sheets 1 inch apart. (IF: Brush with egg or milk for browning.) Bake in a preheated 425 degree oven for 12-15 minutes.

BUT I CAN'T EAT THAT

CHAPTER 3

ITALIAN BREAD
    1 tablespoon sugar
    2 teaspoons salt sense
    2 packages dry yeast
    5 cups flour (all purpose or bread)
    1 tablespoon clarified butter OR Safflower oil
    1 3/4 cup warm water (110 degrees)

    Mix salt, sugar, and yeast with 2 cups of flour. Melt butter and heat water in the microwave. Beat into flour until mixed, 2-3 minutes. Add more flour a little at a time to get a stiff dough for kneading. Knead on a floured board for 10 minutes. Divide in half. Roll out each portion 10x15 inches square and roll it up. Oil the inside of a plastic bag. Put the dough inside the bag and refrigerate overnight. The next day remove dough and slash the top of loaf. Let rise while preheating oven to 425 degrees. Bake 25-30 minutes until hollow sounding when tapped on the bottom of the loaf.

IF: Brush with egg whites on top of loaf before cooking for faster browning.

For **BREAD STICKS**-After rising, cut dough into pieces and roll into long pencil shapes. Place on a greased T-Fal cookie sheet 1 inch apart. Bake in a preheated 400 degree oven for 15-20 minutes. Sprinkle sea salt over top OR brush with butter before cooking.

IF: Brush sticks with egg whites before cooking and sprinkle with Sesame Seeds.

**To add more nutrients and loads of color to bread try these fun additives.

<u>Red</u>-Omit 1 3/4 cup water and proof yeast with 1/2 cups warmed tomato juice at 110 degrees instead. Add in a 12 oz. can of tomato puree with 1 1/2 teaspoon Pizza Herbal Seasonings. Mix into dough when adding flour.

<u>Green</u>- Omit 1 3/4 cup water. Proof yeast with 1/2 cup cooking water from spinach at 110 degrees F. Add in 3/4 to 1 cup spinach puree with 3/4 teaspoons Vegetable Seasonings. Mix into dough when adding flour.

CHAPTER 3

ITALIAN BREAD (Cont.)

Orange-Omit 1 3/4 cup water. Proof yeast with 1/2 cup cooking water from carrots OR carrot juice. Add 3/4 cups pureed cooked carrots with 3/4 teaspoon nutmeg. Mix into dough when adding flour.

Mini instructions for colored loaves.

Mix as above recipes by adding and omitting what is needed. Let rise 1/12 hours, covered in a warm spot. Punch down and make 2 free form round loaves. Place on a greased T-Fal tin. Slash with a razor blade. Cover with a large bowl and let it rise 45 minutes to 1 hour. Bake in a preheated 350 degree oven for 35-40 minutes. Loaf should sound hollow on the bottom when finished baking.

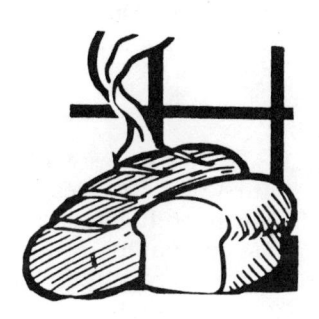

CHAPTER 3

HEAVIER ENGLISH MUFFIN BREAD
2 cups evaporated milk
1/2 cup water
5 cups all purpose flour
2 packages dry yeast
1 tablespoon sugar
2 teaspoons Salt Sense
1/4 teaspoon baking soda

Heat water in microwave until warm (if using probe, program at 110 degrees). Add yeast to warm water. Stir until dissolved. Add sugar and stir and proof yeast 5-10 minutes. In a large bowl whisk flour, salt and baking soda together. Slowly stir in milk and yeast mixture to form a dough. Knead on a floured board 5 minutes or until satiny. Turn into a buttered bowl covering all sides of the dough with butter and cover. Let the dough rise until doubled, 1-1 1/2 hours. Punch down and divide in half, making 2 loaves. Let dough rise again in a buttered loaf pan for 45 minutes to 1 hour. Bake in a preheated 400 degree oven for 25-30 minutes. Loaf should sound hollow when tapped on bottom. Cool on wire rack.

ZUCCHINI BREAD-with Brown Rice Flour
1 1/2 cups plus 2 tablespoons Brown Rice Flour
1 1/4 teaspoon homemade baking powder
1/2 teaspoon baking soda
1/2 teaspoon sea salt
2 large eggs, beaten
1/4 cup clarified butter
1 teaspoon Vanilla Extract (no alcohol)
6 tablespoons fructose
2 tablespoons cinnamon
1/2 teaspoon nutmeg
1 pound of fresh zucchini

Wash and scrub zucchini well. Shred in food processor. Mix all ingredients together, mixing in zucchini last. Bake in a 9x5 inch greased and floured loaf pan. Cook in a preheated 350 degrees oven for 45 minutes to 1 hour.

BUT I CAN'T EAT THAT

CHAPTER 3

ZUCCHINI BREAD
    3 eggs beaten
    1 cup Safflower oil
    3/4 cup fructose
    2 cups grated zucchini (washed well)
    2 tablespoons Vanilla Extract (no alcohol)
    3 cups flour
    1 teaspoon baking soda
    2 1/2 teaspoons homemade baking powder
    3 teaspoons cinnamon
    1 teaspoon Salt Sense

Sift dry ingredients together twice. Set aside. Beat wet ingredients together. Mix grated zucchini with wet mixture. Slowly add in dry ingredients, mixing lightly. Pour into 2 greased loaf pans. Bake in a preheated 350 degree oven for 45 minutes to 1 hour until browned and passes the toothpick test.

IF: You can add 1/4 cup chopped pecans, raisins OR dried fruits to bread before cooking.

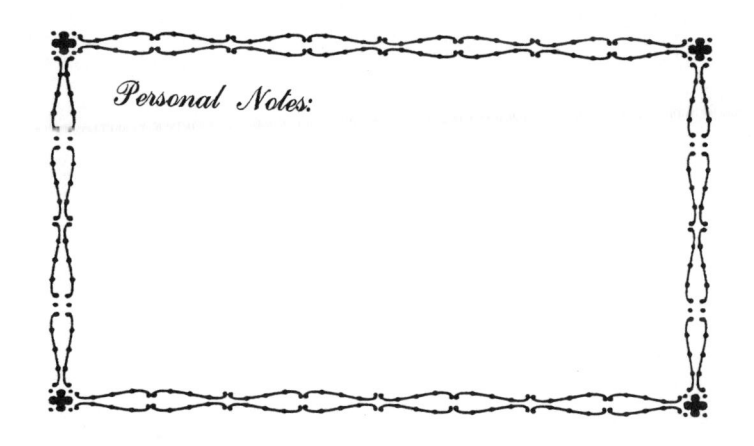

Personal Notes:

BUT I CAN'T EAT THAT

CHAPTER 3

DROP BREAD
    1 1/2 tablespoon dry yeast
    1 cup flour (all purpose OR bread flour)
    1/4 cup warm water
    1 tablespoon sugar
    1/2 teaspoon Salt Sense
    2 cups flour

    Add 1/4 cup warm water (110 degrees) with sugar and salt to yeast. Proof yeast mixture for 10 minutes. Combine yeast with 1 cup of flour. Beat both mixtures together for 3 minutes. Stir in 2 more cups of flour. Drop into a greased casserole dish. Let dough rise for 1 hour, covered. Punch dough down in dish and cover with waxpaper. Let rest 10 minutes. Drop into a greased round casserole dish. Let dough rise for 1 hour. Bake in a preheated 400 degree oven for 35-40 minutes. The casserole makes a nice round loaf. Drop Bread should sound hollow on bottom when done.

IF: Brush with egg whites on top of loaf before cooking for faster browning.

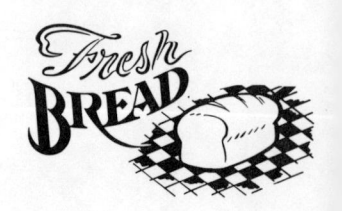

CHAPTER 3

RYE TORTILLAS
    2 cups rye flour
    1/2 cup plus 1 tablespoon cold water
    1/2 teaspoon Salt Sense OR sea salt
    1/4 cup Safflower oil
    lard (no preservative)

Mix all ingredients together. Knead on floured (rye flour) board 5 minutes until smooth and pliable. Shape into a 6 inch log. Cut into 8 equal pieces. Flatten and roll from the center of each piece. Stack on a plate with waxpaper between each tortilla. Covered and chill until needed. Cook both sides in a T-Fal skillet, lightly brushed with lard over medium heat for 1-1 1/2 minutes each side until browned. This tortilla is not flexible and is better served flat. Serve hot with fillings OR serve plain.

RYE ALLERGY LOAF
    1 1/3 cups rye flour mixed with 2/3 cup rice flour
    2 tablespoons fructose
    1/2 teaspoon Salt Sense
    10 teaspoons homemade baking powder
    2 teaspoons Safflower oil
    1 1/3 cup water

Sift dry ingredients together. Add oil and water and mix well. Pour into a greased loaf pan. Bake in a preheated 350 degree oven for 40 minutes. Bakes 1 loaf. This loaf keeps for 2 days. You can omit the fructose. Rye Allergy Loaf is a heavier bread

CHAPTER 3

DROP BISCUITS
    2 cups all purpose flour OR 2 1/4 cups cake flour
    2 1/4 teaspoons homemade baking powder
    1 teaspoon salt sense OR 1/2 teaspoon sea salt
    2 tablespoons butter (non colored)
    1 1/4 cups evaporated milk

Sift all dry ingredients together three times. Cut in butter. Lightly stir milk into dry mixture with fork. Drop on greased T-Fal tin. Bake in a preheated 450 degree oven for 10-15 minutes. Do not over bake. Makes 12 large biscuits. Serve with butter and honey while hot.

CUT BISCUITS
    1 3/4 cup all purpose flour OR 2 cups cake flour
    2 1/2 teaspoons homemade baking powder
    1/2 teaspoon salt sense
    1/3 cup butter OR lard
    3/4 cup evaporated milk OR buttermilk

Sift all dry ingredients together three times. Cut butter into dry mix. Stir in milk with a fork. When dough is soft and easy to roll, knead it slightly into a ball. Shape into a circle 1/2 inch thick. Flour hands and fold three times. Cut into biscuits all the way through the three layers. Place on greased cookie sheet 1 inch apart. Brush with egg OR milk for faster browning. Bake in a preheated 425 degree oven for 12-15 minutes. Cuts 15 biscuits.

CHAPTER 3

BBP BISCUITS

    1 cup all purpose flour
    1/4 teaspoon Salt Sense
    2 1/4 teaspoons homemade baking powder
    1 1/2-2 tablespoons lard OR butter
    1/3 cup water

Sift dry ingredients together. Cut in butter until crumbly. Moisten dough with water. Turn into a floured board and knead 1/2 minute. Roll 1/4 inch thick. Cut with a round, 2 inch cutter. Place 1 inch apart on a buttered baking sheet. Bake in a preheated 400 degree oven for 12-15 minutes. Eat with loads of butter, honey OR jam.

IF: Can substitute milk for water.

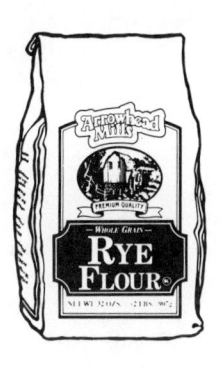

RBP BISCUITS

    1 cup rye flour
    1/4 teaspoon Salt Sense
    2 1/4 teaspoons homemade baking powder
    3 tablespoons butter
    3-4 tablespoons water

Sift dry ingredients together. Cut in butter until crumbly. Moisten with water adding a little bit at a time. Knead 1/2 minute on a (rye) floured board. Roll the dough to 1/2 inch thickness. Cut with round 2 inch cutter. Place biscuits 1 inch apart on a buttered baking sheet. Bake in a preheated 450 degree oven for 15 minutes.

CHAPTER 3

RYE MUFFINS
    1 cup rye flour OR 2/3 cup rye with 1/3 cup rice flour
    2 1/4 teaspoons homemade baking powder
    2 tablespoons fructose
    1/4 teaspoon Salt Sense
    1/2 cup cold water
    2 tablespoons Safflower oil OR clarified butter

Sift all ingredients together. Add water to oil and stir into dry ingredients until lumpy. Put into a buttered T-Fal muffin tin. Bake in a preheated 400 degree oven for 30-35 minutes, until muffins pull away from sides.

IDEA: Substitute 2 tablespoons crushed fruit for 2 tablespoons fructose.
         Substitute 1/2 cup fruit juice for 1/2 cups water.

APPLE MUFFINS
    2 eggs
    1 cup Safflower oil
    3/4 cup fructose
    1 teaspoon Vanilla Extract (no alcohol)
    2 cups all purpose flour
    2 teaspoon cinnamon
    dash of ground clove
    1/4 teaspoon Salt Sense OR sea salt
    1 1/4 teaspoon homemade baking powder
    4 cups chopped apples (4 apples)

Beat eggs for 3 minutes with electric mixer. Add oil, fructose and vanilla flavoring. Sift rest of dry ingredients together. Slowly add this to the egg mixture. Peel, core and shred the apples in a food processor and add to mixture. Put in a greased T-Fal muffin tin. Bake in a preheated 350 degree oven for 20-25 minutes until browned.

IF: 1/2 cup chopped nuts can be added to batter.
        1/2 cup raisins can be added to batter.

CHAPTER 3

PEACH MUFFINS

    2 cups all purpose flour
    3 1/4 teaspoons homemade baking powder
    1/2 teaspoon Salt Sense
    2 eggs
    1 can (8 ounces) peaches in its own juice OR
    3/4 cup peaches drained
    1/4 cup clarified butter

Sift the dry ingredients together. Drain and reserve 1 cup of peach juice and chop peaches. (Add water to make it one scant cup of liquid if not enough juice.) Mix dry ingredients gently together with the 1 cup of juice. Stir until moistened. Place mixture in a buttered T-Fal muffin tin, filling tin 3/4 full. Bake in a preheated 400 degree oven for 20 minutes or until browned.

SWEET PINEAPPLE MUFFINS

These muffins are very sweet.
    2 cups all purpose flour
    3 3/4 teaspoons homemade baking powder
    1/2 teaspoon Salt Sense
    1/4 cup clarified butter
    1 egg, beaten
    1 (8 oz)can crushed pineapple in its own natural juice
    1 teaspoon cinnamon

Sift dry ingredients together. Set aside. Cream butter until light in color with electric mixer. Add egg to the butter mixture, mixing until smooth and light. Add pineapple juice and beat well. Slowly add flour mixture blending in a small amount at a time. Fold crushed pineapple into this mixture. Fill buttered T-Fal muffin tins 1/2 full with batter. Bake in a preheated 400 degree oven for 25 minutes until browned. Serve warm.

IF: Sprinkle fructose and cinnamon over top of muffins before cooking.

CHAPTER 3

RICE MUFFINS
    1 cup all purpose flour
    1/2 teaspoon Salt Sense
    1 1/2 teaspoons homemade baking powder
    2 small eggs
    2/3 cup natural applesauce
    1 cup cooked Brown Sweet Rice OR Sushi Rice
    2 tablespoons butter

    Cook rice adding butter (to rice) while it is still hot. Beat eggs with the applesauce. Sift all dry ingredients 2-3 times. Stir in dry ingredients with rice mixture until all flour is moistened. Fill well buttered T-Fal muffin tins 2/3 full. Bake in a preheated 425 degree oven for 20-25 minutes. Muffins should be browned. Serve hot. To reheat use microwave 15-20 seconds on high, wrapped in a linen or paper towel.

IF: Substitute milk for juice.
      Add 1 tablespoon of fructose for sweeter muffins.

CORN PONE PANCAKES

Large	Small	Ingredients
2 1/2	1/4	cups ground corn meal
1/2	1/4	teaspoon sea salt
1 1/4	1/2	cup water plus 3/4 cup
1/4 cup	2	tablespoons Safflower oil

    Bring water to a boil. Add cornmeal and salt, mixing well. Add oil and 3/4 cup of cold water. Stir until batter becomes stiff. Oil two T-Fal cookie sheets. With an ice cream scooper place dough on sheets and flatten into cakes 3 inches round. Bake 45 minutes in 400 degree oven. For smaller pancakes cook 8-15 minutes. Edges should be browned. Serve hot with butter.

BUT I CAN'T EAT THAT

CHAPTER 3

<u>ZUCCHINI PANCAKES</u> (Egg and Wheat Free)
    2 cups grated (well washed) zucchini
    1 Egg Substitute (Mix: 1 1/2 tablespoon Safflower oil, 1 1/2 tablespoon water, and 1 teaspoon homemade baking powder)
    1/2 cup Tapioca flour
    1/8 teaspoon sea salt

    Mix all ingredients together. Let mixture rest while preheating grill or iron skillet. Make pancakes 2-3 inches. Fry in a little lard, clarified butter OR Safflower oil until crisp on both sides. Inside of pancakes will be soft.

<u>ZUCCHINI PANCAKES</u> (Regular)
    2 cups grated zucchini
    1 beaten egg
    1/2 cup flour
    1 teaspoon homemade baking powder
    1/4 teaspoon Salt Sense

    Mix all ingredients together. Let mixture rest while preheating grill or iron skillet. Make pancakes 2-3 inches. Fry in clarified butter until crisp on both sides. Inside of pancakes will be soft.

<u>FRESH CORN PANCAKES</u>
    2 egg yolks
    2 egg whites
    4 tablespoons Tapioca flour
    1/2 teaspoon Salt Sense
    1 3/4 cups corn cut from cob

    Whisk yolks. Add flour and salt. Next, mix in corn. Beat egg whites until stiff and fluffy. Fold egg whites into mixture. Cook on a preheated grill with clarified butter. Use 1 tablespoon of batter per pancake, flattening with the spatula. Brown both sides. Serve hot.

IDEAS: This is a nice side dish for any meal.
IF: Use all purpose flour instead of Tapioca flour.

CHAPTER 3

AUNTIE'S PANCAKES
1/2 plus 1/8 cup flour
1 1/2 teaspoons homemade baking powder
1 1/2 teaspoon fructose
1 egg
1/2 cup milk (or juice)
1 tablespoon Safflower oil OR clarified butter

Sift all dry ingredients together. Beat egg and add to dry ingredients, then add oil. Do not over mix. Cook on a preheated grill with clarified butter. Brown both sides.

RICE PANCAKES
3/4 cup cooked brown OR white rice
1 cup of your favorite fruit juice
1 tablespoon Safflower oil
1/2 cup flour (rice flour, Tapioca flour OR all purpose flour)
pinch of nutmeg OR cinnamon
pinch of sea salt
2 1/4 teaspoons homemade baking powder
clarified butter OR lard

Mix all ingredients together. Drop batter onto a hot grill or T-Fal pan by tablespoons. Brown both sides.

ORANGE PANCAKES
1 cup flour
1/2 teaspoon homemade baking powder
1/4 teaspoon Salt Sense
2 eggs
1/4 cup Safflower oil OR clarified butter
1 1/2 cups de-acid orange juice

Sift all dry ingredients together. Whisk oil and eggs together. Mix in juice a little at a time with dry ingredients using oil and eggs as a base. Consistency should be like a thick cream. Pour 1/4 cup of batter into a preheated 10 inch T-Fal pan. Spread by tipping pan and smoothing out batter with spatula making a thin crepe. Brown only one side. Roll up to serve. Serve with butter and sprinkle top with powdered sugar, brown sugar OR date sugar.

CHAPTER 3

GREEN PANCAKES
>   2 cups (16 ounce bag) frozen Lima beans
>   1/2 cup Chicken Stock
>   1 Egg Substitute (1 1/2 tablespoons water plus 1 1/2 tablespoons Safflower oil plus 1 teaspoon homemade baking powder)
>   2 tablespoons Tapioca flour
>   dash of salt

Microwave frozen Lima beans for 3 minutes on 40 percent power with no cover and no water. Stir beans. Cook again for 1 1/2 minutes at 40 percent power. Put beans in the <u>food processor</u>. Process until crumbly, 4 seconds. In a <u>blender</u> add the rest of the ingredients and puree until smoother. (It now looks like guacamole.) To make batter pour easily, add 1 tablespoon of oil and blend again. Batter needs to be thin enough to pour very slowly. Add 1 tablespoon of oil more if it is still to thick. Preheat a T-Fal skillet on <u>high</u> with small amount of lard. Spoon batter into small pancakes and turn down to <u>medium high</u> heat. This makes 9-10 pancakes. Serve hot with sea salt OR drizzle Carrot Dressing over top.

IF: Use a real egg instead of the Egg Substitute.

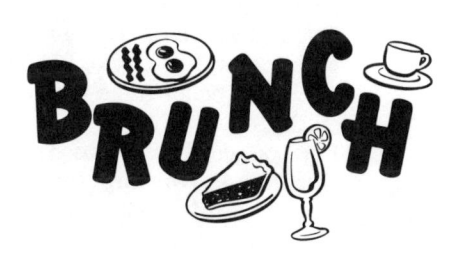

BUT I CAN'T EAT THAT

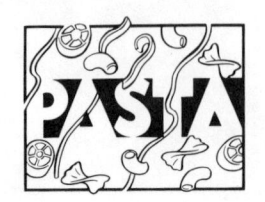

CHAPTER 3
DOUGHS

BASIC PASTA: RAVIOLI
    1 3/4 cup Durham flour
    3 large eggs
    1/2 teaspoon sea salt
    1/4 cup Durham flour for board and rolling

    In the food processor add all ingredients at once, reserving 1/4 cup flour. Process until dough balls up. If dough is too wet add 1 tablespoon of flour at a time. For firmer dough, shape into a ball and cover with a bowl. Let dough rest for a half an hour. For a thinner dough, roll out immediately. Divide dough in half, keeping the dough not in use covered with plastic. Roll out on a floured OR cornstarch dusted board, working from the center out. Roll out a very thin 15x15 inch square. Repeat with the rest of the dough. If using a machine to roll dough out, let dough rest 1/2 hour in a plastic bag first. Don't go past #3 on the hand machine or dough will be to thin. Before cutting, brush off any extra flour. Also spraying lightly with water will improve the stickablity, before adding the top dough. Fill and cover with top sheet of dough. Cut. Let stand at room temperature for 1 hour before cooking. Cooking times vary due to thickness of dough, from 4-10 minutes. Cook in boiling water, keep noodles floating freely. (See Heidi's No Cheese Ravioli for filling.)

IDEAS: Cut leftover noodles into strips for great egg noodles.
VEGETABLE NOODLES:
    For SPINACH NOODLES add 3/4 cup cooked, drained, (squeeze well) chopped spinach, frozen OR fresh. OR use any pureed vegetable I.E.BEETS, CARROTS, TOMATOES each giving its own color.
    Add to all ingredients at the same time.
    Freeze Ravioli individually, then store them together in one freezer bag.
    Use Basic Pasta recipe for noodles. Cut and let dry 1/2 day. Freeze noodles cooked OR uncooked on a cookie sheet then keep in freezer bags for later.
FRIED NOODLES:
    Fry cooked noodles in 375 degree hot oil until golden brown.
IF: Sprinkle Parmesan cheese OR Salt Sense over hot fried noodles and serve.

CHAPTER 3

PASTRY DOUGH
For pot pies
      2 2/3 cups all purpose flour
      1 teaspoon salt sense
      1 cup lard (no preservative)
      7-8 tablespoons cold water

Whisk all dry ingredients together, add lard. Cut mixture into small crumbly pieces with pastry cutter. Add water gently with a fork to make a ball. Divide into six equal parts. Roll into 9 inch circles. Freeze individually or use at once.

IDEAS: Use 1/2 cup lard with 1/2 cup butter for richer tasting crust.

MEAT TURNOVERS:
Stuff with meat puree, fold in half and pinch edges with fork dipped in water. Bake 20-30 minutes in a preheated 375 degree oven.

IF: Add cheese over pureed meat inside meat turnovers.

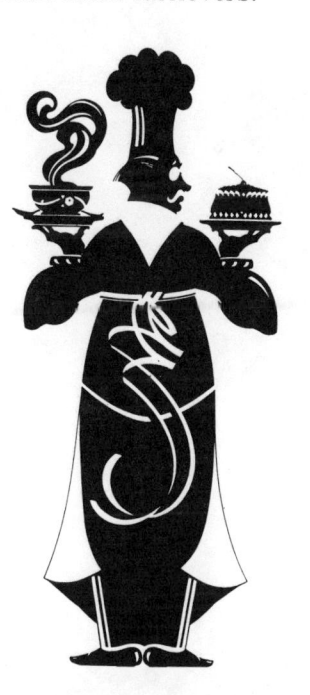

MENU

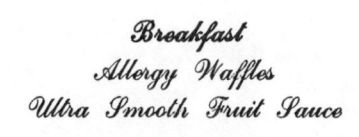

Breakfast
Allergy Waffles
Ultra Smooth Fruit Sauce

Snack
Pureed Meat on
Red Bread

Lunch
Spiced Veal Patty
Quick Broccoli Soup
Brown Rice Cakes

Snack
Customized Granola

Dinner
Fish and Spinach
Homemade Pasta
Boiled Celery
Eatable Short Bread

Snack
Hamburger (Plain)

CHAPTER 3

ALLERGY WAFFLES
1 3/4 cup all purpose flour
2 1/4 teaspoons homemade baking powder
1/2 teaspoon Salt Sense
3 egg yolks
1 1/2 cups natural apple juice
1/3 cup Safflower oil OR clarified butter
3 egg whites
extra oil for iron

Brush waffle iron with extra oil. Preheat waffle iron. Blend all ingredients in large bowl with whisk. Beat egg whites until stiff and fluffy. Set aside. Beat liquids together, except oil, into dry mixture with electric mixer. Do not over mix. When blended add in oil. Fold in the egg whites gently. Pour 1 cup of batter onto a hot waffle iron and close. Cook 3 minutes. Serve hot with butter, Peanut Butter Sauce OR Ultra Smooth Jam.

IDEAS: For a sweeter waffle add 1-3 tablespoons of fructose to dry mixture.

For BLUEBERRY OR FRUIT waffles, add 2/3 cup of fruit to batter before folding in egg whites.

For CAROB waffles add 3/4 cup powdered carob to dry mixture.

For CAROB CHIP waffles add 2/3 cup of carob chips before folding in egg whites. Watch the cooking time on these. The chips melt fast.

IF: For CHOCOLATE waffles add 1/4 cup of cocoa plus 1/4 cup of sugar with dry mixture.

CHAPTER 3

FLOUR TORTILLAS
    2 cups all purpose flour
    1 tablespoon Salt Sense
    6 tablespoons lard (no preservative)
    1 cup water

    Whisk flour and salt together. Cut lard into flour until crumbly. Heat water in the microwave for 50 seconds on high power. Slowly mix hot water to mixture making a soft dough. On a floured board knead dough 5 minutes until smooth and velvety. Cut dough into 3 oz. pieces using kitchen scissors. Roll each piece into a flat tortilla. Keep the rest of dough covered with a damp towel. Roll dough out from the center to the edges. Cook tortillas in a hot iron skillet without any oils. Cook 1-2 minutes per side depending on how thin it is rolled. Tortillas freeze nicely for 2 to 3 months with wax paper in between.

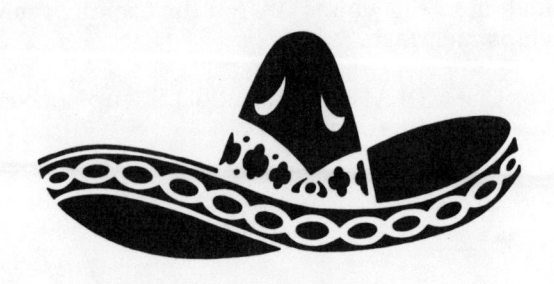

CHAPTER 3

RICE

Rice grains come in many different flavors, textures, colors and smells. Many more appealing than not. Here are some to consider:

<u>Sweet rice</u>;   white short grain and sticky (Sushi)

<u>Sweet brown rice</u>;   brown, short grain, creamy in texture and sweeter in taste

<u>Long white rice</u>;   long grain, good for stir frying

<u>Long grain brown rice</u>;   firmer when cooked, good for stir frying and nice flavor

<u>Koyeco Rose</u>;   white short grain, softer when cooked, slightly sweet, excellent flavor

<u>Basmati rice</u>;   long grain, dark rice with a nutty flavor, firmer

<u>Wild rice</u>;   this is really a grass seed, black in color, usually mixed in combination with other rice, used in stuffings

Combinations of rice are readily available. Here is one good example: Jubilee Blend by Lundberg Farms which contains–Wehani, black japonica, short and medium grain red rice, short and long grained brown rice, plus sweet brown rice. It tastes as good as it looks, so enjoy the different flavors and textures that can be found in this varied grain. Mix them yourself and find your own favorite combination!

White rice needs rinsing before cooking. It is sometimes covered with extra talc or rice flour. (This adds to carbohydrate count and may cause headaches.) Cook all white rice for the same time frames.

<u>BASIC WHITE RICE</u>:   1 cup white rice
                                  2 cups water
                                  Optional: dash of Safflower oil
                                  dash of sea salt

Rinse rice before cooking. Bring water to a boil. Add all ingredients and bring to a boil again. Turn heat down to simmer with a lid for 20 minutes. Remove from heat and let rest for 5 minutes. Do not remove lid during this whole process.

BUT I CAN'T EAT THAT

CHAPTER 3

RICE (Cont.)
The advantage to microwaving white rice is that this method keeps the grains separate. When cooking rice over a burner, the grains tend to stick together. Rinse rice before cooking. Do not add salt or oil when microwaving. Add 1 cup white rice to 2 cups boiling water and cover. Cook on 50 % power for 15 minutes. Remove from heat and let rest for 5 minutes. Do not remove lid during this whole process.

BASIC BROWN RICE:
        1 cup brown rice
        2 1/4-2 1/2 cups water
        Optional: dash of Safflower oil
        dash of sea salt

    Rinse rice before cooking. Add all ingredients together bringing water to a boil. Reduce heat, cover and simmer for 40-45 minutes. Remove from heat and let rest for 5 minutes. Do not remove lid during this whole process.

IDEAS: Try to use a pan with a heavier bottom and a tight lid.
           Rice can be cooked with any broth desired for added flair and taste.
           Minced vegetables can be added to the boiling water.
           Any seasonings can be added to cooking water.
           A tad of oil in the cooking water will help keep the grains separated.

    Most diet requirements for serving rice are 1/2 cup cooked rice. Brown rice is very beneficial to hypoglycemic and Candidas patients. This is due to a slower breaking down period and absorption rate of the complex carbohydrates in brown rice. Brown rice is also higher in protein than white rice.

CHAPTER 3

CROCK POT BROWN RICE
    1 cup brown rice
    3 cups water
    1 teaspoon salt sense

Rinse rice before cooking. Cook all in a Crock Pot for 2 hours on high setting.

IDEA: Cooking in a Crock Pot overnight on low, yields a hot Cream of Rice Cereal in the morning. Or cook in the Crock Pot on low for 8 hours.
    Using above creamy mixture, place in buttered mold and refrigerate over night. Remove from the mold in the morning and slice thin. (Can dust with rice flour first.) Deep fry OR pan fry slices until crispy.
    Use apple juice instead of water and add 1/2 cup of shredded apple just before serving.

IF: Add 1/2 cup of raisins and nuts for a crunchy texture.

READY BROWN RICE
    1 cup sweet and short brown rice
    1/2 cup Koyeco white rice
    3 cups Chicken Stock
    drop of Safflower oil
    1/2 cup minced celery
    1/4 teaspoon curry powder
    1/2 teaspoon onion powder
    1/2 teaspoon celery salt
    sea salt to taste
    dash of turmeric and paprika

Rinse rice before cooking. Mix all ingredients together except the white rice. Bring to a boil. Cover and reduce to low, simmering for 25 minutes. Add rinsed white rice and bring to a boil again. Recover and reduce heat. Simmer 20 minutes more. Remove from heat and let rest for 5 minutes covered. Serve hot.

IDEAS: Add different vegetables to broth.
    Fry unused rice in Safflower oil.
    Make fried rice by adding cooked meats.

IF: For added color mix in red pepper or pimento.

CHAPTER 3

HERBS AND RICE

   3 cups Chicken Stock
   1 cup brown rice
   1 tablespoon onion powder
   dash of garlic powder
   1/2 teaspoon thyme
   1/2 teaspoon chervil OR savory
   1/2 teaspoon sweet basil
   1 Tablespoon parsley
   1 bay leaf

Rinse rice before cooking. Add all ingredients to pan. Bring broth to a boil. Reduce to low, cover and simmer for 40 minutes. Remove from heat and let rest for 5 minutes. Do not remove lid during this whole process. Discard bay leaf. Serve hot.

IDEAS: Mix in wild rice.
         Substitute Lamb Stock for Chicken Stock.

BROWN RICE CAKES

These are great for packing on trips or campouts.
   1 cup brown rice
   1/2 teaspoon sea salt
   2 3/4 cups water
   1 grated carrot
   1 tablespoon onion powder
   1/4 teaspoon ground ginger
   1/4 teaspoon sweet basil
   1/2 cup chopped spinach (cooked and squeezed dry)
   1 tablespoon Safflower oil

Rinse rice before cooking. Add rice to water and bring to a boil. Reduce heat to low, cover and simmer for 60 minutes, adding in carrots the last 20 minutes. When rice is finished cooking add rest of ingredients by hand or in food processor. Process lightly 2-3 times. Do not turn into a paste. Form patties 3 inches round and flatten. Grease with oil a T-Fal cookie sheet. Bake 30 minutes in preheated 350 degree oven. Turn cakes over and cook 20 minutes. The T-Fal will crisp up the surface of the patty. Cool completely before packing. Brown Rice Cakes can go without refrigeration for a day.

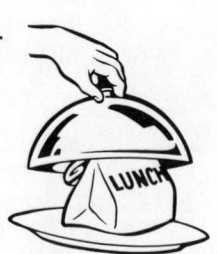

BUT I CAN'T EAT THAT

CHAPTER 3

FRIED "RICE A TUNA"
This fast throw together dish is up to your desecration. If you like more of one ingredient and less of an other add it OR deduct it. Simple mathematics.
- Cooked Short and Sweet Brown Rice (cooked)
- onion powder
- savory
- sea salt
- paprika
- chopped celery
- tuna fish (fresh cooked OR canned)
- Safflower oil

Sauté celery with Safflower oil for 5 minutes until celery is transparent. Sauté rice with celery until rice is browned. Add tuna fish (drained) last and heat through. A great dish served on lettuce with tomato wedges for lunch.

IDEAS: For a little change of pace this makes a good breakfast.

INDIAN WEHANI RICE
Good for breakfast or lunch.
- 1 cup Wehani rice
- 2 1/4 cup Stock OR water
- 1/2 cup cubed cooked chicken
- 1/4 cup crumbled cooked ground veal
- 1/2 teaspoon savory
- 1/2 teaspoon curry
- sea salt to taste
- tad of Safflower oil

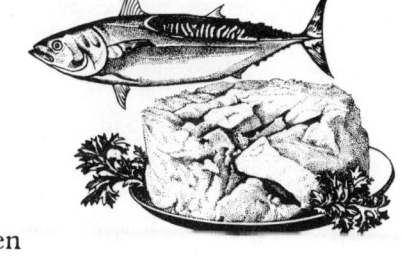

Rinse rice before cooking. Bring rice and stock to a boil. Reduce heat and simmer for 40 minutes, covered. Add meat and all spices for the last 5 minutes of cooking time. Remove from heat and let rest for 5 minutes. Do not remove lid during this whole process. Serve hot.

BUT I CAN'T EAT THAT

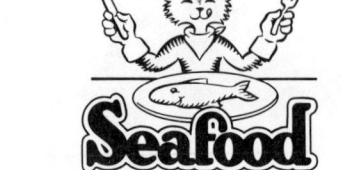

CHAPTER 3

Seafood

INDIAN WEHANI RICE (Cont.)
IDEAS: Serve on a bed of:
- shredded lettuce
- rice macaroni
- rice spaghetti
- Homemade Pasta
- pastry

Use for a stuffing in:
- chicken or turkey cavities
- large shelled macaroni

For lunch add:
- shredded carrots, sweet peas, chopped celery, cooked broccoli.

IF: Sprinkle with Parmesan cheese when rice is hot.
Mix cold Indian Wehani Rice with Hellman's mayo and serve over lettuce with pear slices.

CAPTAIN J.R.'S SEAFOOD SPECIALTY
1 cup cooked Lundberg Jubilee Gourmet Brown Rice
2-3 tablespoons chopped celery
1 tablespoon onion powder
1/2 teaspoon sea salt
1/4 teaspoon sweet basil
1/4 - 1/2 pound cooked filet of perch and halibut
1 tablespoon Safflower oil

Sauté celery in Safflower oil until crisp, 5 minutes. Sauté cooked rice with celery and seasonings. Add sweet peas and sauté with mixture 5 minutes. Add cooked fish only to warm. Serve with Rye crackers on the side.

IDEAS: Add thickened fish stock to all after cooked.
To enhance the fish flavor, precook rice using fish broth instead of water.
IF: Sauté jubilee sliced red pepper along with the celery for color.

CHAPTER 3

SWEET PEACH BREAKFAST RICE
    1 cup cooked brown rice (warm)
    1 (16 oz.) can of peaches in its own juices
    1/2 cup celery
    1/2 teaspoon onion powder
    1/8 teaspoon sea salt
    1/4 teaspoon curry powder
    1/4 teaspoon ground ginger
    1 tablespoon Safflower oil

Chop celery and sauté 5 minutes in oil. Drain peaches and use juice another time. Chop peaches adding spices, then heat with celery. Toss in warm rice last. Serve plain for breakfast.

IDEAS: For lunch serve over a bed of shredded lettuce.

APPLE BREAKFAST DELIGHT
    1/2 cup cooked brown sweet rice (cold)
    1/4 cup homemade Apple Sauce (no sugar)
    1 shredded apple (sweet Red or Golden Delicious)
    dash nutmeg or cinnamon

Combine all ingredients together and serve immediately.

IF: Sprinkle with dried fruits and crushed nuts.

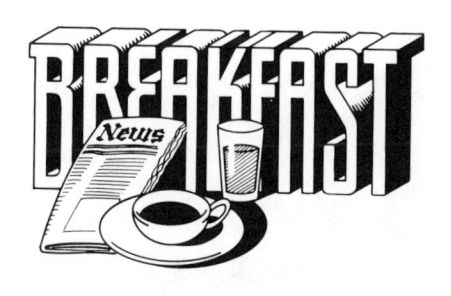

Chapter 4

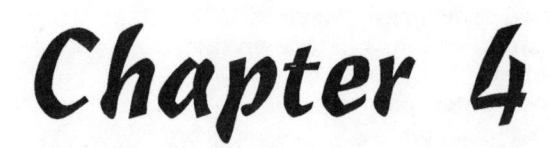

Fruits and Vegetables

Apples

Carrots, Cauliflower, and Corn

Potatoes

Zucchini

Combination Veggies

Steaming Chart

Salad Ideas

BUT I CAN'T EAT THAT

CHAPTER 4
APPLES

Apples are great for dessert and satisfies those "sweet" cravings. Apples are low in "fructose" (sugar) levels and are well tolerated. Some people can tolerate apples cooked but not raw and vice a versa. For mold sufferers, applesauce over 18 hours old should be frozen in individual portions. Here are several methods of cooking applesauce that are time savers.

APPLESAUCE-MICROWAVED
Wash apples with soap and water before using them with the skins on. Roughly cut up 6 apples, peel and remove seeds. Put in a microwavable bowl adding 1/2 cup water OR juice. Cover with plastic wrap. Cook 11-12 minutes stirring once or twice. Put cooked apples through a Foley Food Mill. Reserve liquid to thin out applesauce if needed.

IDEAS: For a sweeter, spicier flavor, add 1/3 cup of fructose, 1/2 teaspoon cinnamon, and 1/8 teaspoon allspice OR 1/8 teaspoon nutmeg after the sauce is made.
Freeze the rest of the apple juice in ice cube tray for Mini Popsicles OR melt the cubes and use in apple pies OR for just plain nibbling.

CROCK POT APPLESAUCE
Clean and cut 2 1/2 pounds of apples. Put in a Crock Pot adding 2 tablespoons apple juice, 1/2 teaspoon pure Vanilla Extract and 1/3 cup fructose. Cover and cook 3 hours on the high setting. Put cooked apples through a Foley Food Mill adding reserved liquid for thinning if needed.

IDEAS: The applesauce liquid is excellent to drink by itself!.
Add 2-3 tablespoons of fructose if needed after cooking.

APPLESAUCE
Wash and cut apples. Fill a dutch oven with cut apples and add 3/4 cup of water. Cover and bring to a boil. Turn heat to low. Simmer for 45 minutes to 1 hour until the knife pierces the apples easily. Put cooked apples through a Foley Food Mill and add reserved liquid to thin sauce if needed.

IDEAS: For an energy saver-put dutch oven in the oven at 350 degrees for 1 hour if your oven is already in use cooking a meal.

BUT I CAN'T EAT THAT

CHAPTER 4

APPLESAUCE TIPS

Experiment with different types of apples when they are in season. Some apples do not need extra sweetening. Personal tastes vary greatly on this. My favorites are Red Delicious and Golden Ozarks.

> Some apples need a longer cooking time depending on how ripe they are.
> For every 4 cups of cooked applesauce add 1/4 cup of fructose if needed OR tolerated.
> Applesauce freezes well for months.
> Left over apple juice can be frozen into great tasting popsicles for quick "sweet tooth attacks".

Spices and/or fruits can be used to change the flavor of applesauce. Try using curry, cinnamon, allspice, raisins, pureed cranberries, pineapples OR other tolerated fruits. Combinations can be limitless.

IF: Honey OR cane sugar can be added to sweeten the applesauce.

APPLE SMOOTHIE

Using the cooked juice from the applesauce you've just made, add:
    1/2 cup apple juice
    1/8 teaspoon ground cloves
    1/8 teaspoon ground cinnamon
    2 apple juice ice cubes
    2 tablespoons Rice Lite drink (or powdered milk)
    2 tablespoons of a banana

In a blender mix all the ingredients together until foamy and serve immediately for a nice cool treat.

BUT I CAN'T EAT THAT

CHAPTER 4

SIMPLE FRUIT SAUCE
    1 cup fruit OR 1 cup berries

Place fruit a in food processor and blend until smooth. Cook in a T-Fal sauce pan, stirring occasionally until fruit boils. Reduce heat and simmer until condensed and thick. Mixture will be sweeter when concentrated. This takes 1 1/2-2 hours. Store in an air tight container in the refrigerator.

    IDEAS: Add 1/2 teaspoon pure Vanilla Extract (no alcohol) when mixture is cooler.

QUICKER SAUCES
    1 can peaches OR a tolerated fruit, packed in its own juice
    1-1 1/2 tablespoons Arrowroot

In a food processor add all ingredients and process until smooth. Cook mixture down on medium heat, stirring constantly until thickened, 10 minutes. Remove from heat. Do not boil. Store in an air tight container in the refrigerator.

APPLE BUTTER (No sugar, No cider)
    1 cup homemade Applesauce (no sweetener added)
    1/2 teaspoon cinnamon
    1/2 teaspoon nutmeg
    1/2 teaspoon allspice

Spice applesauce heavily with cinnamon, nutmeg and allspice. Cook it down for 2 hours on a stove OR 2 to 3 hours in a preheated 275-300 degree oven. Apple Butter will turn brown and become thick. Cool and store in an air tight container in the refrigerator.

JAM FORMULA
    1 1/2 cups of pureed fruit
    1/2 teaspoon Vanilla Extract (no alcohol)
    1 package unflavored gelatin

Dissolve gelatin according to the directions using juice instead of water. Heat fruit in the microwave. Add vanilla. Slowly add gelatin to the hot mixture a little at a time using a whisk until well blended. Cool. Keep refrigerated in an air tight container.

CHAPTER 4

APPLE JELLO
    1 package non flavored gelatin
    1/4 cup unsweetened natural apple juice
    1 3/4 cup unsweetened natural apple juice

Mix gelatin with 1/4 cup juice to dissolve, 3-5 minutes. Boil 1 3/4 cups apple juice in microwave. Add cold gelatin to hot juice. Refrigerate in parfait glasses. Great plain.

IDEAS:
    1/2 cup of shredded apples can be added after the gelatin begins to set.
    1/2 cup of bananas can be added in the same manor, so the fruit does not sink to the bottom.

IF: Add 1/2 cup nuts to garnish the top of gelatin.

APPLE PUFF
    3-4 apples, cored, peeled and shredded
    1/4 cup natural apple juice
    3 tablespoons fructose
    1 Vanilla Bean
    1/2 teaspoon cinnamon
    1/2 teaspoon cream of tartar
    5 egg whites, room temperature

Boil juice adding apples and Vanilla Bean for 8 minutes, covered. Remove bean and discard. Remove pan from heat, add fructose and refrigerate for 10 minutes to cool. Beat eggs with cream of tartar until stiff. Fold into chilled apples. Spoon into a 1 1/2 quart souffle dish. Bake in a preheated 450 degree oven for 15 minutes or until browned. Sprinkle extra fructose and cinnamon over the top of Apple Puff for garnish.

IF: Sprinkle powdered sugar over top if tolerating cane sugar.

CHAPTER 4

FROZEN WATERMELON
Cut watermelon meat out of rind and remove the seeds. Puree in a food processor. Freeze in a shallow pan. Scoop into an air tight container for freezing. Keep frozen until use.

IF: Add fructose to taste before pureeing, but is great tasting served without it.

PEACH BUTTER
2 tablespoons Simple Fruit Sauce (Peach)
1/2 cup butter

Put ingredients into a food processor and blend until butter is light and airy. Chill and serve over pancakes and waffles. This butter improves with age.

IF: Add 1 tablespoon fructose or brown sugar and 1/4 teaspoon lemon juice for sweetness.

FRUIT IDEAS
All these methods work with most fruits and fruit purees.

Fructose can be added if tolerated.

You can use frozen berries and fruits.

You can add fresh chunks of fruit to these homemade jams and sauces.

You can mix several fruits together. For example: apple-pear; peach-apricot; blueberry-cherry.

When using canned fruits, pick fruits in their own juices.

Keep in mind that pineapple and grape juices are higher in sugars. You want to avoid these if you are dealing with Hyperactivity problems.

BUT I CAN'T EAT THAT

CHAPTER 4

CARROTS

Carrots are at their best when homegrown and eaten right out of your own garden. They are second best when store bought at the peak of their growing season. Try to purchase the youngest and thinnest carrots for greater sweetness. The fatter carrots are good for carving decorations, but not so tender for eating.

Sliced carrots are a must for refrigerator munchies, a constant on hand treat and essential for those on diets. They keep well for a week with a little water in the container. On hand carrot snacks are great with Peanut Butter Spread on them, diced and cooked for a last minute dinner vegetable and can fix any salad. For those with new braces; shredded carrots are better.

BAKED SHREDDED CARROTS
4-5 carrots, peeled and shredded

Put in a greased casserole and dot with 2-3 tablespoons of butter. Cover and bake in a preheated 325-350 degree oven for 25 minutes. Sprinkle top layer of carrots with cinnamon and ground clove spice.

IDEA: Top with: 1 tablespoon of butter with 1/4 teaspoon sweet basil and 1 teaspoon parsley.
Use curry powder and ground ginger together and adjust to your liking in melted butter.
IF: Mix 1 tablespoon fresh lemon juice with any of the above butters.

GRATED CARROT SALAD
2 cups grated carrots (peeled)
1/4 cup diced apples
2 teaspoons Safflower oil
optional: sea salt to taste

Mix all ingredients together and serve.

IF: Add chopped raisins and/or nuts.
OR mix in mayo with chopped celery.

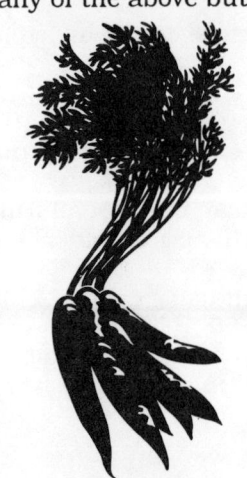

CHAPTER 4

CARROT SAUCE
1 cup shredded carrots (peeled)
1 cup H2O
1/4 teaspoon sweet basil
1/8 teaspoon sea salt
1 tablespoon Arrowroot

Steam or cook carrots in water. Reserve liquid. In a food processor puree carrots with salt, oil, basil and Arrowroot. Heat mixture on medium heat with reserved liquid until thick. Stir often. Puree again to create a smooth sauce.

IDEAS: Substitute 1 cup Chicken Stock with 1 teaspoon curry powder instead of plain cooking water.

SWEET THINS
1 pound carrots, peeled and jubilee sliced
1/2 cup natural apple juice
2 teaspoon Arrowroot
1 1/2 teaspoon clarified butter OR Safflower oil
parsley OR dill

Steam carrots until tender, 5-10 minutes. Mix apple juice with Arrowroot. Cook on medium heat, whisking until thickened. Do not boil. Serve over carrots, topped with butter and garnished with parsley.

CHAPTER 4

CAULIFLOWER

Whole head cauliflower cooked on a decorated platter is simply impressive to guests. This very simple dish is cooked in a microwave, sprinkled with water, wrapped in plastic wrap for 4 minutes in high power. Let stand for 4 more minutes. If steaming, cook for 10 minutes. Cooking in water on stove, covered, cook 10-15 minutes. Preparation for this fun vegetable is carving out the center stem while keeping the florets whole. To wash, soak in salted water until clean. Rinse well. Let head sit to drain.

IDEAS: Sauté cauliflower in oil or clarified butter.
Serve mixed with sweet peas or other vegetable combinations.
Eat raw or cooked, hot or cold in salads.
Dust thinly sliced, cooked, florets with flour and sauté.
Use rice flour OR Tapioca flour with Safflower oil OR clarified butter to sauté with.

IF: When cauliflower is warm, add hot cheese sauce or melt cheese over the top.
Use your favorite batter and deep fat fry cooked florets.

CHAPTER 4

CORN

When corn on the cob is in season, it is great! Select cobs having smallish kernels for the sweetest taste. Large kernels tend to be starchy tasting. Boil in water for 10-15 minutes. Serve with clarified butter. To use up leftover corn, (only one day old, please) strip from cob and freeze for future use in recipes such as Smashed Corn and Corn Pancakes.

SMASHED CORN

Put 4 cups cooked corn in a food processor then through a Foley Food Mill. Heat before serving. Whisk 2 tablespoons clarified butter into corn over medium high heat until corn thickens. Serve hot and steamy.

CORN PANCAKES
    1 large egg
    1 cup fresh corn (from cob)
    1 tablespoon Tapioca flour
    1/4 teaspoon sea salt
    Safflower oil and clarified butter for cooking

Mix all ingredients together (except oil and butter) with an electric beater. Fry up 1 tablespoon of batter at a time in skillet with 1/2 Safflower oil and 1/2 clarified butter. Brown 3-4 minutes each side. Drain and serve warm. These pancakes freeze well.

IF: Use all purpose flour.
       Can add 1 teaspoon fructose to the batter.

CHAPTER 4

POTATOES

If you are restricted on your carbohydrates, potatoes must be watched carefully due to their starch level. One serving of a potato per meal is recommended for those on a low carbohydrate diet.

POTATO CAKES
1 large peeled and finely shredded potato
1 beaten egg
1 1/2 tablespoon Tapioca flour
1/4 teaspoon sea salt
1/2 teaspoon onion powder
butter and Safflower oil for cooking

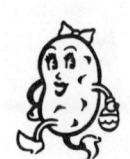

Combine all ingredients. Mix well. Use a mixture of half butter and half Safflower oil in a heavy cast iron pan for cooking. Drop potato mixture by tablespoons and flatten with fork. Brown both sides. Drain and serve hot with salt.

IDEAS: Serve with homemade Applesauce.
IF: Serve with sour cream.
            Use all purpose flour instead of tapioca flour.
            Add in fresh grated onions instead if onion powder.

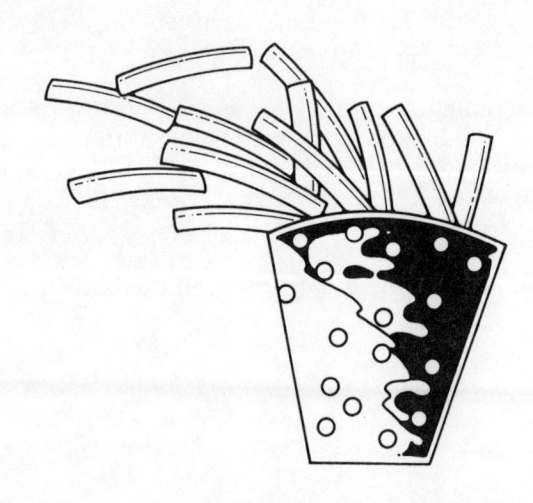

CHAPTER 4

POTATO CHIPS

Peel potatoes and slice into very thin chips. Soak in cold water for 30 minutes to remove excess starch. Drain and dry on cloth towels. Add 1 tablespoon of Safflower oil to a T-Fal cookie sheet. Cook one layer of chips at a time. Bake in a preheated 425 degree oven for 10 minutes (total time), flipping chips over the last 5 minutes. You can cook the fries with OR without Safflower oil on the bottom of the pan. Salt while hot with sea salt OR onion salt.

POTATO CROUTONS

Make baked potatoes in the microwave oven OR use leftover potatoes baked in the oven. Peel and dice potatoes into the size of small croutons. On a T-Fal cookie sheet, melt 2 tablespoons butter and 2 tablespoons Safflower oil. Roll all sides of potato squares in oil. Broil at 400 degrees, 5 minutes each side. Total time 10-15 minutes. Blot on paper towels and serve hot.

IDEAS: Sprinkle paprika, onion powder OR garlic powder over potatoes before cooking.
Potato Croutons are great with meals, as snacks and on salads.

IF: While potatoes are hot, toss with Parmesan cheese.

PLAIN BAKED POTATOES

Wash potatoes and prick skins with a fork. Oil skins with Safflower oil if you like the skins to stay soft. If you like crustier skins, cook plain. Bake in a preheated 400 degree oven for 1 hour or until they are squeezable. (Use pot holders for this test.)

IDEAS: Serve baked potatoes with clarified butter sprinkled with paprika.
Pour beef chips in brown gravy over top of opened potato for a meal.
Add a chicken sauce with chunks of chicken over top of opened baked potato.
Mix cooked lamb, turkey and veal with cooked vegetables in a Chicken Stock White Sauce, over top of opened baked potato.

IF: Serve dollops of sour cream over top.
Scoop out cooked potato, leaving 1/4-1/2 inches of potato meat inside the skins. Butter the potato meat before melting different cheeses over top of opened skins, under the broiler.

BUT I CAN'T EAT THAT

CHAPTER 4

FRIES

There are many different french fry cutters on the market now that are really fun to use. These are great for the picky eaters in the family. Snacks after school can be curly fries, shoestring potatoes, criss cross, cottage fries or steak fries. Peel and slice potatoes into desired shapes. Soak in ice cold water at least 30 minutes to remove excess starch. Drain and dry on cloth towels. Fry small batches at a time, so hot oil doesn't cool down too fast for the next batch. (This produces soggy fries.) Good frying oils to use (if tolerated) are: Pure Corn oil, pure Peanut oil and pure Safflower oil. Lard (no preservative) can be used also.

Chips–Fry 10 slices at a time for 2–2 1/2 minutes.

Sticks–Fry 8–10 pieces at a time for 3 1/2–4 minutes.

Thick Wedges–Fry 2 minutes, cool for 10 minutes. Refry 8–9 minutes. I call this method fry and refry. Refrying crisps up the outside. This works with the stick fries also, but keep an eye on them carefully. You may want to shorten up the first frying time.

SKILLET HASH BROWNS

Peel and shred potatoes. Preheat a cast iron skillet on medium high heat with half Safflower oil and half clarified butter. Add potatoes and flatten out like a pancake. Cook until bottom is brown, for 10 minutes. Cut in half and flip over keeping Hash Browns in tact. Brown the other side. Add more oils if potatoes stick to skillet. Season to taste with: sea salt, paprika, onion powder, celery powder, garlic powder OR any of your favorite unlimited combinations.

IDEAS: Add beaten eggs over top the of Hash Browns after one side is browned.
Add cooked meats to shredded potatoes before cooking.
Add sautéd chopped celery before cooking.
IF: Add onions, peppers and mushrooms to shredded potatoes before cooking.
Add sausage, lunch meats and top with cheeses.

Combinations are up to your diet, imagination and tastes. This is a great protein meal for breakfast. Skillet Hash Browns can be served any time.

CHAPTER 4

ZUCCHINI

BROILED ZUCCHINI

Wash skins of zucchini thoroughly with <u>soap</u> and <u>water</u> to dispel any mold. Rinse well and dry. Slice zucchini into thin 1/4 inch slices. Add 2 tablespoons Safflower oil to a T-Fal cookie sheet. Coat zucchini with oil on both sides. Broil zucchini at 400 degrees for 10 minutes. Turn zucchini over and broil 5 minutes more. It's naturally sweet and great served plain. You can season with onion powder, garlic powder, celery salt, sea salt or paprika before or after cooking.

IF: Broiled zucchini can be served in tomato sauce.
        Sprinkle Parmesan cheese over top before serving.

ZUCCHINI CAKES

Use shredded zucchini for tender and very delicate tasting pancakes. These are much softer and are not as crispy as the potato cakes.

    1 large peeled (finely shredded zucchini)
    1 beaten egg
    1 1/2 tablespoon Tapioca flour
    1/4 teaspoon sea salt
    1/2 teaspoon onion powder
    A mixture of half clarified butter and half Safflower oil for cooking

Wash skins of zucchini thoroughly with <u>soap</u> and <u>water</u> to dispel any mold. Combine all ingredients and mix well. Use a mixture of half clarified butter and half Safflower oil in a heavy cast iron skillet. Drop mix by tablespoons and flatten with fork. Turn pancakes when brown. Blot on paper towels and serve hot with salt.

IDEAS: Serve with butter and sea salt.
IF: Substitute all purpose flour instead of Tapioca flour.
        Grate one small onion or a couple scallions into the batter.

MICROWAVED ZUCCHINI

Wash skins of zucchini thoroughly with <u>soap</u> and <u>water</u> to dispel any mold. Slice or dice zucchini. Place in a microwavable bowl adding 2 tablespoons water OR stock. Cover and cook on high power 5-6 minutes, stirring once. Let stand 3-4 minutes.

CHAPTER 4

YOUR FAVORITE VEGGIES WITH CURRY
    1 cup Chicken Stock
    1 tablespoon Arrowroot
    2 1/2 teaspoons curry powder
    1/4-1/2 teaspoons sea salt
    2-3 tablespoons Safflower oil
    4 to 6 different vegetables of your choice

Select 4 to 6 of your favorite veggies, sliced, diced shredded OR julienne cut. (After washed and peeled.) Heat Safflower oil in a Wok. Stir fry all vegetables for 5-10 minutes, stirring constantly. Remove veggies from Wok. Whisk stock with Arrowroot and curry powder and add enough stock to cover veggies. Stir until stock thickens then add cooked vegetables. Season with sea salt to taste.

IDEAS: Can substitute 1 tablespoon Tapioca flour for Arrowroot, but remember that Tapioca flour needs more cooking time than Arrowroot.
    Vegetables that you can use are carrots, sweet peas, zucchini, squashes, green beans, cauliflower, Mung beans, water chestnuts or bamboo shoots. Use 1 cup of stock, but change flavors and seasonings;
    For Beef Stock use 1 teaspoon sweet basil.
    For Veal Stock use 2 teaspoons Bouquet Garni.

IF: Green or red pepper, broccoli, precooked Brussels sprouts and skinned tomato pieces without seeds.

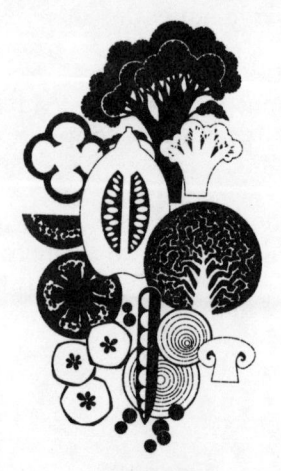

CHAPTER 4

STIR FRY BOK CHOY WITH NAPA CABBAGE
2 pounds Bok Choy
1 head of Napa cabbage
4-5 tablespoons Safflower oil
1/2 teaspoon sea salt
1/2 cup Chicken Stock
2 tablespoons Chicken Stock
1/2 tablespoon Arrowroot/OR Tapioca flour
Safflower oil for cooking
Optional: 1 teaspoon fructose

Wash and cut Bok Choy in one inch sections. Wash and spin dry Napa cabbage and shred. Heat oil in Wok on medium high heat. Stir fry Napa until slightly wilted. Remove and put aside. Stir fry Bok Choy in Wok with more oil if needed for 5 minutes. Add Chicken Stock with Bok Choy and simmer 5 minutes more. Whisk 2 tablespoons cold Chicken Stock with Arrowroot until dissolved. Add thickening mixture to Wok with Napa cabbage. Stir until thickens. Do not boil. (If using Tapioca flour add more time for thickening.) Serve as a side vegetable.

CREAMY SPINACH
1 package frozen chopped spinach
1 cup Chicken Stock
1 tablespoon Arrowroot
1/2 tablespoon onion powder
1/4 teaspoon sea salt

Cook spinach, drain and squeeze well. Combine all ingredients except spinach in pan. Cook over medium heat until stock thickens. Add spinach to heat through.

IF: Serve with a dot of butter OR sour cream over top.

BUT I CAN'T EAT THAT

CHAPTER 4

CELERY IDEAS
Wash and cut into julienne strips. Keep in the refrigerator with a little water for snickelsnackles any time.

Chop celery in food processor. Sauté celery in a T-Fal pan with water OR fry in an iron skillet with Safflower oil. Keep in freezer for later use in meat loafs, hot salads, rice, stuffing, etc. (This is a great time saver.)

Serve Herbal Vegetable Sauté over hot celery.

STEAMED CELERY
Wash and slice celery. Boil water in a steamer. When steam is escaping from the sides of the pan, add celery and cover. Turn heat down to medium high heat and steam 15-18 minutes.

MICROWAVE CELERY
Wash and slice celery. Cook celery in a microwavable casserole with 2 tablespoons water OR Vegetable Stock, covered. Cook 5-7 minutes stirring once. Let rest 5 minutes.

BOILED CELERY
Wash and slice celery. Add celery to boiling water OR stock. Cover and cook over medium high heat for 10 minutes. Remove quickly when done.

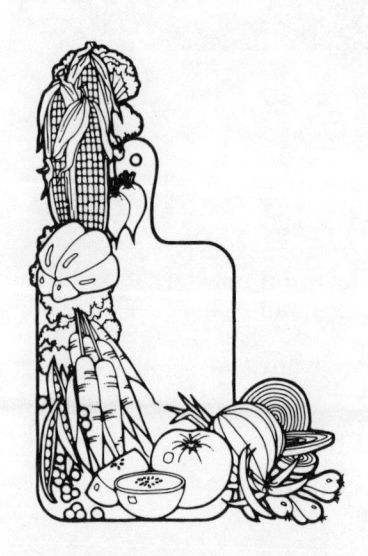

CHAPTER 4

CELERY STUFFING
1 cup cooked rice (brown OR white OR wild rice)
3/4 cup chopped celery
1/4-1/2 teaspoon sea salt
1 tablespoon onion powder
1/8 teaspoon thyme

Sauté celery for 5 minutes with water in a T-Fal skillet OR use oil in an iron skillet. Mix all ingredients together and stuff any thing you like.

IDEAS: Serve Celery Stuffing as a side dish.
Good stuffed in a flank steak.
Good stuffed under chicken breast skin. (Loosen skin up with your fingers first, then stuff.)
Good stuffed inside a turkey.
Good for stuffing pork chops.
IF: Substitute bread crumbs plus an egg, for rice.
Add real onions to celery and sauté.

HERBAL VEGETABLE SAUTE
Serve over hot vegetables like carrots, green beans, sweet peas, cauliflower and celery.
1 tablespoon Safflower oil
1 tablespoon clarified butter
2 tablespoon chopped parsley
2 tablespoons chop chives
1 tablespoon sweet basil
1/2 tablespoon onion powder

Mix all together and use when sauting precooked vegetables. (Leftovers are good also.)

IF: Use olive oil and margarine instead of Safflower and butter.
Add 1/4 teaspoon oregano and 1/4 teaspoon garlic powder to spice list in recipe.
Can add a chopped tomato with skins off and seeds removed.
To make a <u>marinade</u> from this add lemon juice OR gluten and yeast free vinegar to lightly steamed vegetables overnight and serve cold. (This keeps for one day only.)

CHAPTER 4

STEAMING VEGGIES TIMETABLE

Broccoli florets and stems	10 minutes
Brussels Sprouts (whole)	15 minutes
Carrots (whole baby)	5 minutes
Carrots, sliced	7–10 minutes
Cauliflower, whole	15 minutes
Cauliflower, florets	10 minutes
Celery, diced	15 minutes
Corn on Cob	15 minutes
Green beans, whole	15–20 minutes
Green Peas, fresh	8 minutes
Potatoes, white, quartered	20 minutes
Spinach	10 minutes
Zucchini, sliced	5 minutes

Steaming broccoli florets and cauliflower florets can taste tough if outer skin is not peeled off the stems first. A potato peeler works great. A skinless broccoli stem may be steamed this way and tastes similar to water chestnuts. Try it!

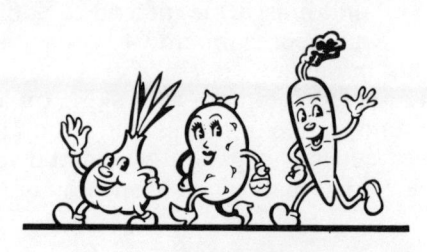

CHAPTER 4

SALAD IDEAS
Ingredients to have on Hand:
- Lettuce-Iceberg, Bib or Boston
- Cooked OR steamed vegetables
- Cooked meats, fish and poultry
- Cooked rice-brown, white, sweet and wild
- Fresh raw veggies
- Cooked rice noodles, rice spaghetti, rice shells and rice elbow noodles
- Canned meats, poultry, fish (packed in water)
- Mixed cut fruits
- A safe salad dressing of Safflower oil with sea salt is quite tasty.

Cut, slice, dice or shred vegetables and proteins and add to noodles. Mix and arrange handsomely on a platter. Garnish with elected seasons: sweet basil, savory, tarragon, dillweed, parsley, paprika.

IDEAS: Hot rice is great on cold lettuce!
IF: Try gluten and yeast free vinegar mixed with Safflower oil for dressing.
Add cooked Quinta, nuts, cheese, artichoke hearts, avocado, cooked eggs, commercial salad dressings, lemon juice OR tomato juice with spices.

SALAD DRESSING FOR FRUITS
This non-allergenic fruit dressing can be poured over fruit salads of mixed peaches, apples, bananas, grapes, strawberries, blueberries OR raspberries.
- 1/2 cup of a natural fruit juice
- 1 tablespoon Arrowroot

Whisk juice with Arrowroot and heat until thickens. Do not boil. Cool in the refrigerator, then pour over fruit salad.

SHREDDED CARROT SALAD
Make Salad Dressing for Fruits using natural apple juice and cool. Shred carrots for the base salad instead of lettuce. Chop some raisins and celery and mix all together tossing with dressing.

BUT I CAN'T EAT THAT

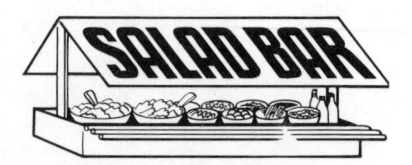

CHAPTER 4

ONE MEAL SALAD
This is especially good if you have a summer garden!
    In a large salad bowl fill half way with hand torn lettuce of your choice. Add shredded carrots and shredded zucchini. Slice up raw green beans, fresh sweet peas (no pods please) and cooked cauliflower florets. Add 1-1/2 cups of steamed, cubed chicken breast, beef, pork or tuna. Toss in 1/2 cups of hot brown rice. Serve with Safflower oil and sprinkle with sea salt for a scrumptious low-cal one dish meal. Garnish with savory and fresh chives.

IDEAS: Squeeze fresh lemon juice over salad.
IF: Use your favorite commercial salad dressing.
                You can add shredded cheese over top of salad.
                Add chopped hard boiled eggs.

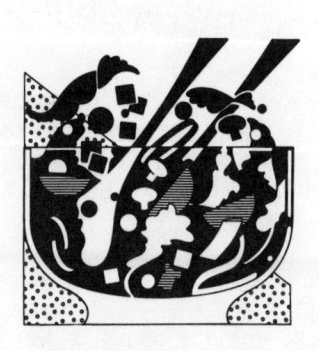

Chapter 5

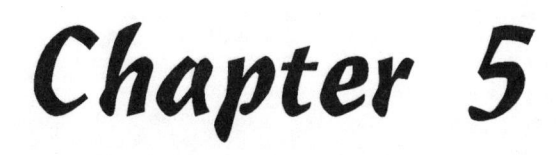

Soups

Seasonings

Sauces

Miscellaneous

CHAPTER 5

SOUPS

People's tastes for soups vary greatly. When using these recipes keep in mind that for thinner soups use more liquid, for thicker soups use less liquids.

BASIC: CHICKEN STOCK

    2-3 pounds of chicken bones (left over carcass, wings, breast bones, cooked and uncooked.)
    8 cups water
    2 teaspoons sea salt
    2 tablespoons onion powder
    1/4 cup parsley
    1 cup chopped celery with tops

    Fill stock pot almost to the brim with bones. Add water to cover bones. Slowly bring to a boil. Skim foam off that forms on top of the water. Mix in rest of ingredients and reduce to low. Cover and simmer for one hour. Remove meat from bones and keep refrigerated for adding later to soup. return bones to stock, cooking for one more hour or until full flavor develops. Cook stock without the lid to reduce and concentrate flavor. Add more sea salt if needed. Strain soup, add meat and refrigerate overnight. Remove covering of fat that hardens on top of the stock and discard. Divide into one or two cup portions and package for freezing. Stock is ready to use as soup bases or sauces. Freeze several ice cube trays for quick mini sauces.

    IDEAS: To vary flavor of stock, mix in veal bones.
                  Add a chopped carrot to sweeten stock.
                  Keep tasting stock as it is cooking until you get the flavor you are looking for. Stock can cook up to eight hours and still have flavor!
                  (But the meat needs to be removed from the bones sooner.)

<u>Quick Cooking Idea</u>-To cook stock in a pressure cooker, use 5 cups of water for 15 minutes after you reach the correct pressure. Let the pressure drop on its own.

BUT I CAN'T EAT THAT

CHAPTER 5

BASIC: BEEF STOCK (OXTAIL)
    3-4 pounds of oxtail bones
    8 cups water
    2 tablespoons sea salt
    2 tablespoons onion powder
    1/4 cup parsley
    2 bay leaves
    1 teaspoon marjoram
    1 teaspoon Bouquet Garni
    1 cup chopped celery with tops

    Brown bones in a preheated 450-475 degree oven for 1/2 hour. Deglaze drippings on bottom of pan with stock for flavor and color.
    Fill stock pot almost to the brim with bones. Add water to cover bones. Slowly bring to a boil. Skim foam off that forms on top of the water. Mix in rest of ingredients and reduce to low. Cover and simmer for two hours. Remove meat from bones and keep refrigerated for adding later to soup. Return bones to stock, cooking for one more hour or until full flavor develops. Cook stock without the lid to reduce and concentrate flavor. Add more sea salt if needed. Strain soup, adding meat then refrigerate overnight. Remove covering of fat that hardens on top of stock and discard. Divide into one or two cup portions and package for freezing. Stock is ready to use as soup bases or sauces. Freeze several ice cube trays for quick mini sauces.

IDEAS: To vary flavor of stock, mix in veal bones.
             Add a chopped carrot to sweeten stock.
             Keep tasting stock as it is cooking until you get the flavor you are looking for. Stock can cook up to eight hours and still have flavor! (But the meat needs to be removed from the bones sooner.)
IF: Add before cooking:
             A chopped tomato or two.
             1 tablespoon Kitchen Bouquet and 1/2 teaspoon Worcestershire Sauce.
             Whole cloves.

Quick Cooking Idea-To cook stock in a pressure cooker, use 6 cups of water for 15 minutes after you reach the correct pressure. Let pressure drop on its own.

CHAPTER 5

BASIC: LAMB STOCK
This is my favorite. Lamb Stock has the most interesting flavor of all the stocks.

    2-3 pounds lamb shanks, bones, shoulders and any left-over roast leg bones (cracked)
    8 cups water
    1 tablespoon sea salt
    2 bay leaves
    1 teaspoon marjoram
    1 teaspoon thyme
    2 tablespoons onion powder
    1 cup chopped celery with tops

Fill stock pot almost to the brim with bones. Add water to cover bones. Slowly bring to a boil. Skim foam off that forms on top of the water. Mix in rest of ingredients and reduce to low. Cover and simmer for 1 1/2 hours. Remove meat from bones and keep refrigerated for adding later to soup. Return bones to stock, cooking for at least one more hour or until full flavor develops. Cook stock without the lid to reduce and concentrate flavor. Add more sea salt if needed. Strain soup, adding meat then refrigerate overnight. Remove covering of fat that hardens on top of stock and discard. Divide into one or two cup portions and package for freezing. Stock is ready to use as soup bases or sauces. Freeze several ice cube trays for quick mini sauces.

IDEAS: When serving, add steamed julienne carrots and/or sweet peas for color and variety.

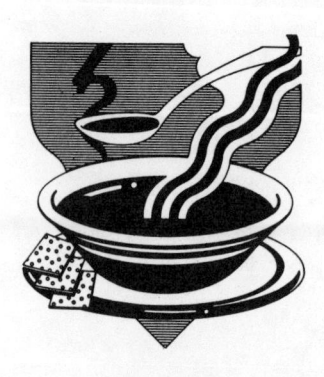

BUT I CAN'T EAT THAT

CHAPTER 5

SOUPS

Once your stocks are made and ready on hand, the soups and sauces made from these bases are up to your imagination. Here are some ideas to get you started...

BASIC: VEGETABLE BROTH

1 pound of fresh vegetables to every 2 1/2 cups of Chicken Stock. Use celery, green beans, Lima beans, potatoes, carrots, cauliflower, cabbage, tomatoes OR any left-over veggies. Add 1 teaspoon thyme and parsley. Add more sea salt if needed. Dice vegetables before cooking for a fuller taste. Bring broth to a boil, skim if needed, cover and reduce to low heat. Cook 45 minutes. Strain and serve hot. Garnish with cooked vegetable florets.

IDEAS:

THICKER VEGETABLE SOUP
Puree vegetables cooked in Vegetable Broth through a Foley Food Mill. Add 1/2 cup of pureed cooked rice to thicken.

CHUNKY VEGETABLE SOUP
Add fresh (OR frozen) whole OR sliced vegetables to broth. Cook 10 minutes. Serve hot.

LITE LETTUCE SOUP
This is extraordinarily tasty!
1 head of lettuce (Iceberg or Boston)
sea salt
1 2/3-2 cups Chicken Stock

Clean and discard center of lettuce and shred. Add lettuce to broth and bring to a boil over medium heat. Skim if needed, cooking for 30-45 minutes. Puree in a food processor until smooth. Serve hot with fresh cut chives as a garnish.

CREAM OF LETTUCE SOUP
Puree 1/2 cup cooked brown rice with a small amount of Lite Lettuce Soup. Whisk to incorporate rest of Lite Lettuce soup, adding small amounts at a time.

IF: Serve dotted with real butter melting on top, giving a marbled effect.

CHAPTER 5

VEGETABLE BROTH IDEAS (Cont.)
People's tastes for soups vary greatly. When using these recipes keep in mind for thinner soups use more liquid, for thicker soups use less liquid.

QUICK BROCCOLI SOUP
1 1/2 cups broccoli (frozen for speed, fresh for taste)
1 cup Vegetable Broth
1 teaspoon Vegetable Seasoning
sea salt

Clean, cut (peel stems with carrot peeler if fresh) and cook broccoli in broth. Strain and puree broccoli in food processor slowly adding broth. Serve hot, garnishing with cooked broccoli florets.

CREAM OF BROCCOLI SOUP
Puree 1/2 cup cooked brown rice with a small amount of Quick Broccoli Soup. Whisk to incorporate remaining Quick Broccoli Soup, adding small amounts at a time.

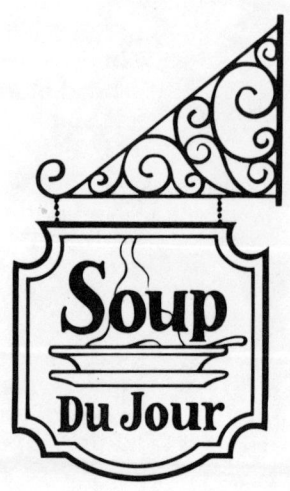

CHAPTER 5

BASIC: ANYTHING GOES SOUP
    1 cup any left-over combination of meats from roasts, meat loaf, hamburger, chicken
    1 cup any left-over carbohydrates noodles, rice OR potatoes
    1 cups any left-over combination of vegetables, carrots, green beans, zucchini, etc.
    Your favorite spices
    3 cups of any flavor Stock or Broth

Bring broth to a boil. Add all spices, then carbohydrates to broth warming thoroughly. Add meat and vegetables last, heating only long enough to warm all ingredients. Serve immediately. This is a complete and nutritious meal in a bowl. Do not reheat.

IF: Add tomatoes for color.
           Use beans, legumes and lentils.

FISH BROTH
This is a delicate fish broth that uses the Vegetable Broth recipe as a base.
    1 1/2 pounds fish (Sole OR Cod) use frame and head of fish, but no gills
    1/2 teaspoon salt sense
    1 tablespoon onion powder
    3 1/2 cups Vegetable Broth

Add all ingredients to pan and bring broth to a boil. Skim foam off that forms on top of the water. Cover and cook for 30 minutes. Strain well with cheesecloth and discard parts of fish. When serving, reheat with fresh raw fish to be served in or with the soup. Cook 8 minutes. Fish Broth freezes well.

IDEAS: This broth is great thickened with Arrowroot for a sauce to pour over baked or sautéd fish fillets.

BUT I CAN'T EAT THAT

CHAPTER 5

CHICKEN STOCK IDEAS

People's tastes for soups vary greatly. When using these recipes keep in mind for thinner soups use more liquid, for thicker soups use less liquids.

CREAM OF CHICKEN SOUP
Bone chicken breasts and poach in Chicken Stock for 4-5 minutes. Remove chicken from stock and dice. Puree 3 cups of cooked brown rice (OR sweet rice) with 1/2-1 cup of Chicken Stock. (Adjust desired thickness.) Return soup to stove and reheat. Add diced chicken, diced cooked carrots and sweet peas to soup. Heat thoroughly. Serve with a sprig of parsley or fresh cut chives.

CELERY SOUP
Add 2 cups chopped celery with tops to 1 1/2 cups Chicken Stock. Cook for 30 minutes and strain. Serve clear OR puree celery and add to soup.

CREAM OF CELERY SOUP
Puree 3 cups of cooked brown rice (OR sweet rice) with 1/2-1 cup of celery broth. Reheat and serve.

SPINACH SOUP
Puree one (9 oz.) package of frozen spinach (microwave and drain). Using a food processor puree spinach slowly adding 1 1/2 cups of broth. To thicken more, use 2 tablespoons Arrowroot. Heat over medium high heat, stir constantly until soup thickens. Do not boil. Garnish with a fresh spinach leaf.

CREAM OF SPINACH SOUP
Puree 3 cups of cooked brown rice (OR sweet rice) with 1/2-1 cup of spinach soup (adjust to desired thickness).

IF: Garnish with a dollop of sour cream over top and a pat of butter.

CHAPTER 5

BASIC:CAULIFLOWER SOUP
    1 head of cauliflower
    1 1/2 cups Chicken Stock
    1 teaspoon Chicken Seasoning
    sea salt

Clean, cut and cook cauliflower in Chicken Stock. Strain and puree cauliflower in the food processor adding stock slowly with the machine running. Soup should be smooth. Serve hot, garnishing with small cauliflower florets sprinkled with fresh tarragon.

IDEAS: For a different taste, add 1/2-1 teaspoon of curry powder to soup.
IF: Garnish with butter.

ZUCCHINI SOUP
    3 large zucchini
    salt sense
    3 tablespoons Safflower oil
    1 1/2 cups Chicken Stock
    dash of nutmeg
    1 tablespoon parsley
    2 jars (4 1/2 oz.) Beach-Nut Stage One Green Beans
    sea salt

Wash, peel and shred zucchini in food processor. Lightly sprinkle Salt Sense over shredded zucchini. Set aside in a colander to drain in the refrigerator for 1 hour. The salt will pull the water out of the zucchini. When zucchini is ready, squeeze all water from it by hand. (Get your kids to do this. They think this is fun!) Reserve liquid. Sauté zucchini in Safflower oil 5-10 minutes. Add reserved liquid and Chicken Stock, bringing all to a boil. Pour into blender adding spices and green beans. Puree until thick, adjust salt if needed. Reheat to serve. Top with fresh chives.

IF: Garnish with a dollop of sour cream OR butter.

BUT I CAN'T EAT THAT

CHAPTER 5

BASIC: SWEET PEA SOUP
    1 bag (16 oz.) of Green Giant sweet peas
    1 1/4 cup of Chicken Stock OR Vegetable Broth

Bring stock to a boil in the microwave. Add peas to hot soup, cooking 3 minutes. In a food processor, process all until smooth. Add 1/2 cup cooked sweet peas to hot soup when serving. Garnish with a couple of fresh mint leaves.

IDEAS: For a more exciting flavor which thickens up this sweet tasting soup, add 1 jar (4 1/2 oz.) of Beach Nut Stage 2 Green Beans when blending.

IMPERIAL GREEN SOUP
    1/2 cup chopped spinach, cooked and drained
    1 jar (4 1/2 oz.) Beach-nut Stage 1 Royal Imperial Carrots
    1/2 cup Chicken Stock
    pinch of sea salt

Add all ingredients to a food processor and puree for 2 minutes until velvety. Reheat in microwave for 3 minutes until hot. Serve with rice cakes.

IF: Good topped with butter.

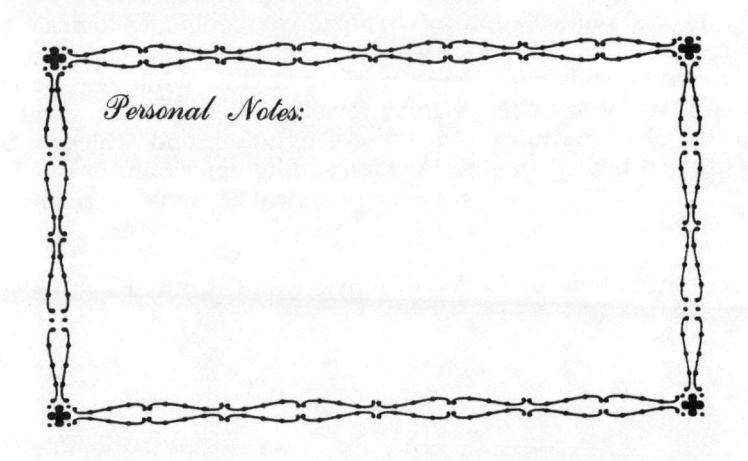

Personal Notes:

BUT I CAN'T EAT THAT

CHAPTER 5

SAUCES

GRAVIES

Gravies can enhance many meats, fish and poultry dishes, turning plain flavors into succulent treats. The key to flavorful gravy is the pan drippings. (My son Jonathan, calls this burnings, not drippings.) Here's where it all starts. With stock and the right thickener for you, even a hamburger can have its own rich sauce.

BASIC: PAN DRIPPINGS

    3 tablespoons fat (from roast, lard, butter OR Safflower oil)
    2 cups cold Stock OR water
    3 tablespoons Arrowroot, Tapioca flour OR rice flour
    sea salt

    Dissolve pan drippings on bottom of roaster with desired liquid. Make a roux with thickener and fat. Slowly add liquid to roux, stirring until gravy thickens. If using Arrowroot, add it to 2 oz. of <u>cold</u> liquid, shaking until dissolved. Slowly add Arrowroot mixture to warm gravy, stirring constantly until thickened. Do not boil. Add sea salt if needed.

IDEAS: Use Fish Stock for fish, Chicken Stock for chicken and pork and (oxtail) Beef Stock for beef when making gravies.

CHAPTER 5

SEASONINGS

Do not over look testing the possibility of molds in dry seasonings. Some may be O.K., while others will bother you. Some fresh herbs will bother you while the same dried herbs won't. Allergies are crazy! Try testing the differences in brands also. This sounds like a large task. Rightly so. But it's only needed to be determined once. Then your cooking pleasures are assured. Here are some suggestions, but don't be afraid to concoct your own special combination! Use seasonings for salads, soups, dips, stews, eggs and more.

DRYING HERBS IN MICROWAVE
Put 1/4 cup fresh garden herbs, washed and dried between two sheets of white paper toweling. Heat on high power for 2-3 minutes until herbs are crumbly. Package in an air tight container.

BEEF SEASONING
Mix together:
- 2 tablespoons dried oregano
- 1 tablespoon dried thyme
- 1 tablespoon paprika
- 1/2 teaspoon sea salt

IF: Dash of black pepper

CHICKEN SEASONING
Mix together:
- 1/4 teaspoon garlic powder
- 1/4 teaspoon onion powder
- 1/4 teaspoon thyme
- 1/4 teaspoon poultry seasonings
- 1/4 teaspoon sweet basil
- 1/4 teaspoon paprika
- 1/4 teaspoon parsley
- 1/4 teaspoon sea salt

IDEAS: Turn seasonings into breading by adding 1/4 to 1/2 cup (dried homemade) French bread crumbs.

CHAPTER 5

PIZZA SEASONING
Mix together:
- 2 tablespoons dried sweet basil
- 1 tablespoon dried marjoram
- 1 tablespoon dried oregano
- 1 1/2 teaspoons dried rosemary
- 1 1/2 teaspoons dried savory
- 1 1/2 teaspoons dried thyme
- 1/2 teaspoon onion powder
- 1 teaspoon dried sage (optional)

Put into food processor and grind into a fine powder.

VEGETABLE SEASONING
- 1 small carrot
- 2 tablespoons dried savory
- 2 tablespoons dries tarragon
- 2 tablespoons dries parsley
- 1 tablespoon dried celery leaves
- 2 tablespoons dried dillweed (optional)

Peel carrot, discarding skins, completely strip the carrot to the core with peeler (or a fine grater). Dry in a 200 degree oven for 1 hour until crumbly. Blend all ingredients together in food processor.

IF: Add 1 tablespoon caraway seed
    1 tablespoon cumin seed
    1 tablespoon coriander seeds

FISH SEASONINGS
- 1 teaspoon dried sweet basil
- 1 teaspoon celery salt OR seed
- 2 teaspoons dried marjoram
- 2 teaspoons dried thyme
- 2 teaspoons dried rosemary
- 4 teaspoons dried savory

Use in a pepper mill. This is also good on a pork roast!

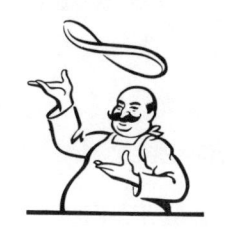

CHAPTER 5

HERBAL BUTTER
Good on chicken.
> Basic: 1/2 teaspoon dried herbs
> 4 tablespoons clarified butter OR Safflower oil
> pinch of sea salt

Use your choice of herbs: chives, sweet basil, savory, parsley, thyme, tarragon OR marjoram. Add herbs to warmed butter and pour over cooked foods.

IF: Use fresh lemon juice instead of sea salt.

SESAME BUTTER
> 1/4 cup clarified butter OR Safflower oil
> 1 tablespoon sesame seeds
> 1/4 teaspoon onion powder
> pinch of sea salt

Add herbs to warmed butter and pour over cooked foods.

IF: Add 2 tablespoons fresh lemon juice plus 1/8 teaspoon grated lemon rind to butter.
Add 1/4 teaspoon garlic powder OR freshly minced garlic to butter.

HERBAL SALT
> 1/3 cup dried sweet basil
> 1 tablespoon sweet basil
> 1/3 cup dried crushed chervil
> 1 tablespoon dried savory
> 1/3 cup dried parsley
> 1/2 tablespoon onion powder
> 1/4 cup sea salt OR 1/2 cup Salt Sense

Add all ingredients to a food processor, blending for 1 minute. Stir down once and blend 1/2 minute more. Put into a shaker.

CHAPTER 5

CHIVE SAUCE
For chicken
>   1 cup Chicken Stock with 1 tablespoon Arrowroot
>   2 tablespoons freshly chopped chives

Mix all ingredients together in small sauce pan. Whisk constantly over medium heat until thick. Do not boil. Serve over chicken, garnish with extra chives.

PEANUT BUTTER SAUCE
Use over homemade waffles and ice cream.
>   1/4-1/2 cup homemade Peanut Butter
>   1 tablespoon butter OR clarified butter

Add ingredients to small glass bowl. Microwave for 30 seconds on high power. Stir. Cook 30 seconds more on high power. Sauce should be liquefied. Spoon over food while hot.

PEACH SAUCE
>   1 can (8 1/4 oz.) Cling peaches in its own juices
>   1 tablespoon Arrowroot

Put all ingredients in a food processor. Turn on and off three times to mix. Process continually for 1-2 minutes until smooth. In a shallow sauce pan whisk peach mixture on medium high heat until thick, for 5 minutes. Do not boil. Serve hot over foods. This is great on German Pancakes OR homemade waffles. Does freeze well, but when reheating in the microwave use 80% power.

IDEAS: Add 1 teaspoon curry powder to sauce before cooking.
Reserve some peaches to add later after the sauce is cooked for a chunky sauce or for a garnish.

CHAPTER 5

PEAR SAUCE

    1 can (8 1/4 oz.) Bartlett pears in its own juices
    1 tablespoon Arrowroot
    1/4 teaspoon cinnamon
    2 tablespoons butter or clarified butter

Put all ingredients in food processor. Turn on and off three times to blend. Process continually for 1-2 minutes until pears are smooth. In a shallow sauce pan whisk pears on medium high heat until thickened for 5 minutes. Do not boil. Serve hot over foods.

IDEAS: Reserve some pears to add later after the sauce is cooked for chunky sauce or for a garnish.

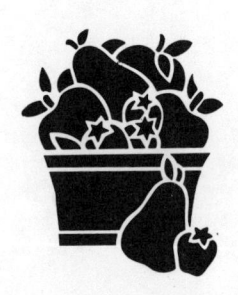

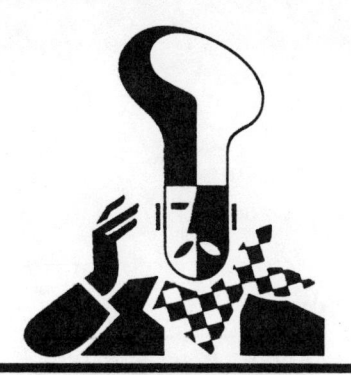

MENU

Breakfast
Banana Dream Shake
Veal Patty (Plain)

Snack
Allergy Waffle
Peanut Butter Sauce

Lunch
Use Pork Roast in
Quick Beef Meal Ideas
w/ Veggies and Rice
Pop

Snack
Potato Cakes

Dinner
Allergy Spaghetti Sauce
over Homemade Basic Pasta
Italian Bread
Herbal Vegetables Sauté

Snack
Crispy Chicken Slices

CHAPTER 5

ALLERGY SPAGHETTI SAUCE

No MSG, preservatives or sugars in the sauce–just great taste. This recipe requires a Crock Pot and a Food Processor.

- 2 cans (16 oz.) Contadina tomatoes
- 1 can (29 oz.) Contadina tomato puree
- 3 cups shredded carrots (use thinner, sweeter carrots)
- 2-3 tablespoons onion powder
- 1 celery rib plus leaves
- 1/4-1/2 cup parsley
- 1/4-1/2 cup Beef Stock
- beef bones
- 1 teaspoon sweet basil
- 1/2 teaspoon thyme
- 1-2 bay leaves
- 2 teaspoons Salt Sense
- dash black pepper
- 1/4 cup Minute Tapioca
- 1/2 minced garlic clove OR 1/2 teaspoon (optional) garlic powder

Chop celery and sauté vegetables in Beef Stock. Add to crockpot with all ingredients except the Tapioca. Cook covered on the high setting for 1 hour in the Crock Pot. Stir and recover. Cook 2 1/2 hours on high setting. Stir in tapioca in the last hour. After cooking remove bones and bay leaves and discard. Puree small amounts of sauce at a time in food processor until smooth and see no seeds, 3-4 minutes per batch. Serve plain or add Meatballs or crumbled Pork Sausage. Adjust salt to taste. Sauce freezes well. When doubling recipe, cook for 2 hours longer. Freeze in ice cub trays for fast extras on tacos, in hamburgers or over zucchini.

IDEAS: If there is an allergy to ketchup, this Sauce is nice for dipping French Fries in.

CHAPTER 5

MISCELLANEOUS

<u>CARROT DRESSING</u> (For Salads)
    1 small jar (4 1/2 oz.) Beach-Nut Stage One Carrots
    1 tablespoon Safflower oil
    3 teaspoons fructose
    pinch of sea salt

Mix all in blender. Serve over salads. Keeps refrigerated for 2 days only.

<u>CROUTONS</u>
    1/4 cup clarified butter
    2 teaspoons herbs (your own favorites)
    4 cups cubed homemade French Bread

Mix and toss all together. In microwave, on white paper toweling, cook 4-5 minutes on high power. Stir several times. As croutons cool, cubes will crisp up. Store in an air tight container.

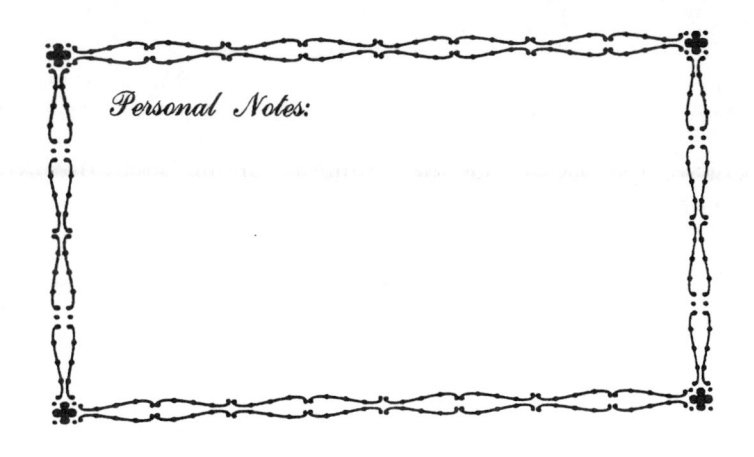

Personal Notes:

CHAPTER 5

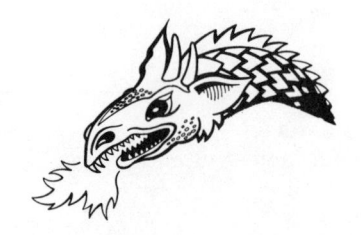

DRAGON COOKIES
Treats for man, boy and his dog (and a good protein source).

When trying out a new treat for our dog, (who also has food allergies) I discovered my son and husband were eating the dog's cookies while they were cooling on the racks. I told them the treats were for our dog and we all had a good laugh. But they still keep eating them every time I make a batch. They really are quite nutritious, good for snacks and training dogs.

    2 large eggs
    3 tablespoons of a sweetener; fructose, honey, molasses, OR brown sugar (all bets went to the molasses)
    1/4 cup Safflower oil
    1/4 cup whole milk
    1 cup rolled oats
    3/4 cup wheat germ
    1/4 cup flour
    1/2 cup currants

    Mix ingredients in mixer one at a time, slowly. Drop by the teaspoon on lightly greased T-Fal cookie sheet OR use a sheet of parchment paper underneath. You can form the dough into round cookies or long sticks. Watch the timing closely for small drop cookies. Bake in a preheated 350 degree oven for 7 minutes on one side then turn cookies over and cook for 7 minutes on the other side. Turn the oven off, open the oven door and keep cookies in the oven 1 hour longer. Omit the 1 hour in the oven after cooking for softer cookies for the human part of the family.

CHAPTER 5

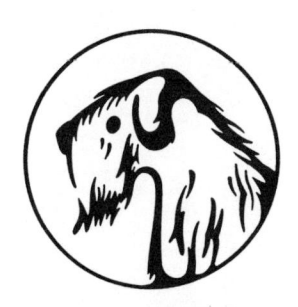

CORNMEAL DROPS
This (no preservative) treat is for your furry friend.
- 1 1/2 cups cornmeal
- 1/2 cup bran flakes
- 2 tablespoons oatmeal
- 2 tablespoons Safflower oil
- 3 cups of Chicken Stock

Mix dry ingredients together. Boil stock then add all ingredients. Let cool. Form into shapes wanted (round or sticks). It's a good idea to flour your hands first before shaping dough. Bake on a greased T-Fal cookie sheet in a preheated 375 degree oven for 20 minutes. Cool and store in the refrigerator or freeze.

A Helpful hint for a sick dog, is to make a batch of Chicken Stock, remove the fat and cook 2 cups with 1 cup of rice. This is just what the Vet. ordered. Use until your dog is better and you can slowly add in his regular food. This is also "safe" for dogs with allergies.

CHAPTER 5

BASIC DRINKS
POP
  1 part sparkling water
  2 parts your favorite juice

Mix and serve over ice with a mint leaf inside the glass.

FRUIT SHAKE
  1/2 cup juice
  1/2 cup fruit
  3 frozen fruit cubes

Puree in blender. Serve over ice and garnish with a mint leaf.

BANANA DREAM SHAKE
  1 banana
  2 tablespoon to 1/4 cup natural apple juice
  1 scoop Vanilla Rice Dream

Puree all in blender. Serve immediately.

IDEAS: This freezes well. Make popscisles in freezer for a cool treat on a hot day.
IF: Use Vanilla ice cream instead of Rice Dream.

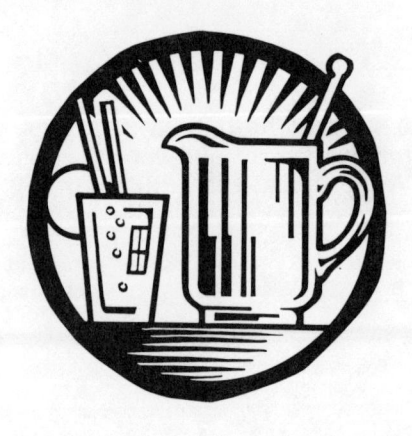

CHAPTER 5

MICROWAVE HINTS

POWER

100%	For cooking meat, good for chicken and fish. Never reheat on high power.
80%	Use for reheating.
50%	For roasting less tender cuts of meat. (20 minutes per pound) Use baking soda on meats as a natural meat tenderizer.
30%	For defrosting, this is a valuable cooking mode for people with mold allergies, where most foods are frozen after cooking. A good power to use with Arrowroot. IF: Use when cooking baby calves liver.
20%	Use as a Crock Pot slow cooking mode. (But do not use the same Crock Pot cooking times).
10%	For raising Bread-place 3 cups boiling hot water in microwave, under the bread. Cover and let dough rise for 20-25 minutes, letting dough rest for 20 minutes.

1. Always let foods <u>rest</u> after microwaving to complete cooking. Calculate half the cooking time for resting.

2. To cook <u>one</u> hamburger, use the <u>browning plate</u> preheated and cook 45-50 seconds at 100% power. To cook one hamburger on a <u>plain microwavable plate</u>, cook 90 seconds at 80% power.

3. To cook <u>one</u> chicken breast (bones in) cook 150 seconds at 100% power. Turn over and cook 150 seconds at 100% power. Let rest for one minute.

BUT I CAN'T EAT THAT

CHAPTER 5

MICROWAVE HINTS (Cont.)

4. To Poach one chicken breast (with bones), boil chicken in 1/2 cup Chicken Stock for 4-5 minutes at 100% power.

5. To make ZUCCHINI for stuffing: Wash well and pierce several times. Cook 4 large zucchinis 7-8 minutes on 100% power turning half way through. Rest 5 minutes. Split and scoop out seeds and add filling, sauce and toppings. Reheat 1-2 minutes on 80% power.

6. For CLARIFIED BUTTER: Microwave 1 pound of butter (cut into 4 quarters). Heat on medium high until melted. Do not boil. Skim off top foam and discard bottom residue. Use clear middle liquid. Stored covered. Do not refrigerate.

IF:
GRILLED CHEESE SANDWICH
Preheat a microwave browning dish. Cook sandwich for 30 seconds on 70% power, uncovered. Turn over and cook 30 seconds more on 70% power.

For COOKING NUTS in a regular oven:
Preheat to 250 degrees:
Almonds	40 minutes
Cashews	40 minutes
Pecans	30 minutes
Peanuts (Unshelled)	25 minutes
Peanuts (shelled)	45 minutes
Sunflowers seeds	20-25 minutes

CHAPTER 5
COOKING TIMES OVER CHARCOAL for a different taste.
Use the electric starter instead of lighter fluid. Lighter fluid may be a culprit to headaches and stomach aches. Important to test this theory out first.

FOODS	RARE	MEDIUM	WELL
Steaks			
First side (1"thick)	2 minutes	4 minutes	5 minutes
Second side	3 minutes	4 minutes	6 minutes
Hamburgers (plain)			
First side	2 minutes	3 minutes	3 minutes
Second side	2 minutes	3 minutes	3 minutes
Hamburgers (stuffed)			
First side		4 minutes	6 minutes
Second side		5 minutes	7 minutes
Lamb Patties			
First side	not recommended	3 minutes	4 minutes
Second side		4 minutes	6 minutes
Fish in pan (covered)		10 minutes, no turning	

Baked potatoes (in foil)
Put potatoes on rack OR right into the coals if camping, turn over in 30 minutes, total time 60 minutes.

Corn
Remove corn silk and soak in water <u>in their husks</u> for 1 hour prior to cooking. Cook corn wrapped in foil, still in their husks, on top of the grill OR put corn into the coals when camping. Grill 1/2 hour turning several times.

Chicken
It's a good idea to boil chicken in water for 10-15 minutes first. This ensures chicken will be cooked thoroughly. Cook on a grill for 30 minutes turning every 10 minutes.

Meat Shish Kabobs
Cook 15-20 minutes, turning twice.

CHAPTER 5

QUICK COOKING TIMES
(Pressure Cooker) for vegetables. All times are cooled at once.

VEGETABLE	ADD WATER OR STOCK	MINUTES
Broccoli, florets	1/2 cup	2
Brussels Sprouts	1/2 cup	3
Carrots, whole	1 cup	8
slices	1/2 cup	2
Cauliflower, whole	1 cup	5
florets	1/2 cup	2
Celery	1/2 cup	2
Corn on the Cob	1/2 cup	3
Green Beans	1/2 cup	3
Lima Beans	1/2 cup	2
Peas, fresh, shelled	1/2 cup	2
Potatoes, whole	1 1/2 cups	15
slices	1/2 cup	3
Spinach	1/2 cup	3

Chapter 6

Sweetmeal Toppers

CHAPTER 6

SWEETMEAL TOPPERS

To find a dessert recipe without cane sugar in it is difficult. In this chapter <u>all</u> dessert recipes are without cane sugar. They contain natural sweet ingredients OR in some cases fructose.

The key word in this chapter is limit. <u>One</u> serving is better than <u>none</u>. One is better (having no reaction from one) than eating 2 to 3 servings and becoming ill. <u>Control</u> is extremely hard when these sweets taste so good. Test these recipes on yourself before you go all out. You may be able to eat some of one recipe and more of another. GOOD LUCK!

<u>APPLES</u>

Baked fruits are great. Apples for one, are sweetest at the peak of their season. Golden Delicious, Golden Ozarks and Rome Beautys are good for baking whole, making apple sauce and homemade Apple Pies. These types of apples have more flavor and are naturally sweeter, requiring no added fructose or cane sugar.

Facts on Apples:
One pound of apples makes 3 cups of sliced apples.

Two pounds of apples makes 3 cups of applesauce or pie filling for one 9 inch pie.

Four small apples equals one pound of apples.

Three medium apples equals one pound of apples.

Two large apples equals one pound of apples.

A peck of apples equals 10-12 pounds of apples.

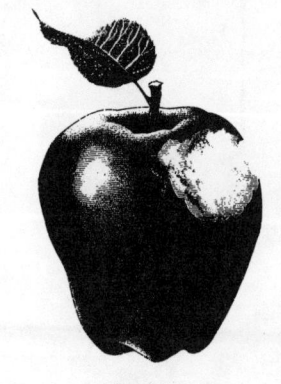

CHAPTER 6

BAKED WHOLE FRUIT
    6 fresh whole fruits (apples, pears, peaches)
    <u>Fruit fillings</u> can be: chopped nuts, dried fruits, nutmeg, canned
        fruit chunks, fresh cut fruits, pureed OR mashed fruit
        1 teaspoon fructose
        cinnamon to taste
        clarified butter
        sprinkle of all spice.

    Wash and peel fruit. Mix all ingredients together. Cut the top 1/4 inch off the fruit. Core and remove the seeds without cutting through the bottom of the fruit. Spoon Fruit fillings inside OR cook plain. Wrap the fruit in foil 3/4 the way up. Bake until tender in a preheated 350 degree oven for 30-45 minutes for peaches and pears, 45 minutes to 1 hour for apples. Serve hot.

BASIC: <u>APPLE LEATHER</u> (Snack)
    Finely shred two pounds of peeled apples. Flatten into a thin layer on a buttered T-Fal cookie sheet. Bake in a preheated 225 degree oven until <u>dry</u>. Approximately 8 hours. Remove carefully from oven and cool. Break into large pieces for better storage. Store refrigerated in an air tight container.

IDEAS: Before baking, sprinkle cinnamon and/or fructose over the top before baking.
              Mix shredded apples with pureed peaches, then flatten and cook.

CHAPTER 6

ALLERGY PIE PASTRY
    2 cups all purpose flour
    1 teaspoon homemade baking powder
    (Sift: 2 teaspoons cream of tartar, 2 teaspoons Arrowroot,
    1 teaspoon baking soda. Measure given amount needed.)
    1 teaspoon salt sense
    1/2 cup lard (no preservatives)
    1/2 cup cold water plus 1 tablespoon if too dry

    With a wire whisk blend flour, salt and baking powder together. Cut in lard with a pastry cutter OR two knives until mixture resembles small peas. With a fork, gently mix in water to make a dough. If dough is too dry, add 1 tablespoon of water at a time, as needed. Do not over work the dough! Roll out 1/2 of the dough between two sheets of wax paper. Use immediately OR freeze until needed. Refrigerate for a half hour if it is too soft to release from wax paper (in warmer weather). Place dough into a pie pan, pricking all over with a fork. Fill with fruit and bake. To bake crust alone, cook at 400 degrees for 10-12 minutes.

To MICROWAVE: use a glass pie pan and cook 10 minutes on high power, rotating the pan once during cooking. Brown for 15 minutes in a preheated 425 degree oven to crisp top of pie. Allergy Pie Pastry freezes well for six months. Extra pastry is great for cut outs and decorations when chilled firmly. Use pastry for individual tarts and pot pies.

IF: Substitute Crisco for lard.

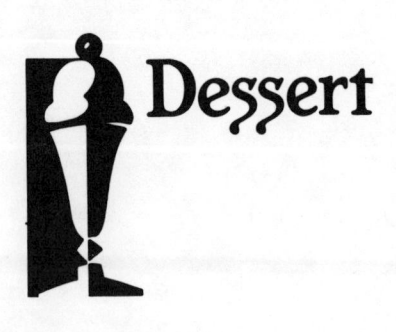

Dessert

CHAPTER 6

ALLERGY APPLE PIE
1 recipe Allergy Pie Pastry
5 to 6 large Red or Golden Delicious apples (OR Rome)
2 1/2 tablespoons Minute Tapioca
1/2 teaspoon cinnamon
dash of nutmeg
1 1/2 tablespoons clarified butter
1 teaspoon Vanilla Extract (no alcohol)

Prepare pastry crust. Roll out on wax paper to fit the bottom of a glass pie pan. Refrigerate the top crust. Peel, remove the seeds slicing apples thin with a food processor. Toss apples with the rest of the ingredients except butter. Let apples sit for 15 minutes to soften Tapioca. Fill pie crust with the apple mixture after pricking pastry bottom well. Dot with butter. Cover with top crust. Prick and design pastry as you wish.

To **MICROWAVE**: Cook for 5 minutes on high power, rotate pan, cook 5 minutes more on high. Remove and place in a preheated 425 degree oven for 10-15 minutes until browned.

To **OVEN BAKE**: Cook in a preheated 425 degree oven for 15 minutes. Turn down to 325 degrees. Cook 30-45 minutes more. Serve warm or cold. Preparation time approximately 1 hour. You can freeze the pie before baking it for two months. To cook frozen pie: Cook in a preheated 450 degree oven for 20 minutes, then turn oven down to 375 degrees for 1 hour or until done.

IDEA: Mix 2-3 tablespoons fructose into the apples.
             Make individual tarts.
             Serve Rice Dream over the top (non dairy ice cream).

IF: Brush egg wash over top pastry crust (1 egg with 1 teaspoon water) for better browning.
             Add 1/2-1 tablespoon of lemon juice to apple filling.
             Serve with ice cream.
             Add 2/3 cup brown sugar to apple filling.

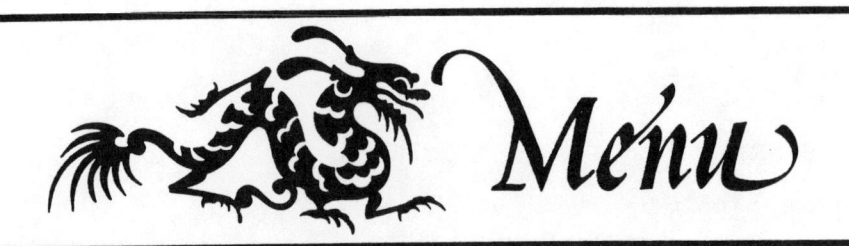

Menu

Breakfast
Chicken Burgers
Skillet Hash Browns

Snack
Fruit Shake
Dragon Cookies

Lunch
Fish Steaks
Indian Wehani Rice
Apple Jello
Grated Carrot Salad

Snack
Peach Muffin

Dinner
Beef Chow Mein
Basic White Rice/Fried Pasta (Homemade)
Allergy Strawberry Pie

Snack
Chicken Stock w/
Chicken and Rice

CHAPTER 6

ALLERGY STRAWBERRY PIE
    1 baked Allergy Pastry Shell
    1 quart fresh strawberries
    3/4 cup fructose
    2 1/2 tablespoons Arrowroot
    Pinch of sea salt
    1 cup distilled water

Wash and hull strawberries. In the food processor, puree 1 cup of strawberries and set it aside.

Combine the rest of the ingredients in sauce pan. Whisk fruit mixture over low to medium heat until thickened. DO NOT BOIL. Stir often for 7-10 minutes and add pureed strawberries. Remove from heat. Arrange whole (or cut) strawberries on bottom of the baked pie shell. Pour the hot fruit mixture over the top of the cut strawberries. Chill in refrigerator at least 5 hours before serving. Serve the same day or one day after.

IDEA: Make individual tarts.
            Serve with Rice Dream on top. (non dairy ice cream)
IF: Serve with whipped cream on top.

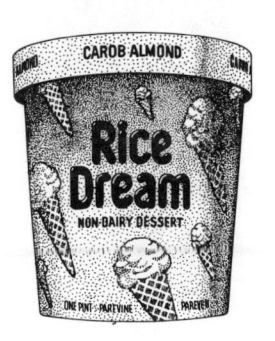

CHAPTER 6

<u>ALLERGY PEACH PIE</u>
This is very rich. Small slivers of pie should be served.
    1 recipe Allergy Pie Pastry
    3 pounds (OR 6 cups, cut) fresh ripe peaches
    3 tablespoons Minute Tapioca
    Dash of nutmeg and ginger
    1 1/2 tablespoons butter
    1/4 tablespoons Vanilla Extract (no alcohol)

Prepare Allergy Pie Pastry. Roll pastry out in between two sheets of wax paper and fit bottom of the pie pan. Prick pastry with a fork. Refrigerate top crust or make lattice slices.

Peel, pit and slice peaches. Toss peaches with all the ingredients except butter. Let for 15 minutes to soften the Tapioca. Put the filling in the pie pan and dot with butter.

Cover the top with the pastry crust OR design a lattice weave. Bake in a preheated 450 degree oven for 15 minutes. Turn the oven down to 325 degrees and cook for 20-25 minutes longer until peaches are soft.

IDEA: Individual tarts are nice.
           Sweeten with 3-4 tablespoons of fructose.
IF: Use Almond Extract instead of Vanilla Extract.

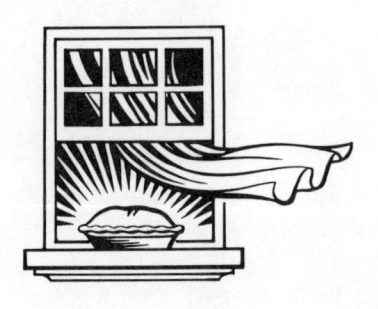

CHAPTER 6

LITE ALLERGY PUMPKIN PIE
    1 baked Allergy Pie Pastry
    1 tablespoon Knox Unflavored Gelatin
    1/4 cup cold water
    4 egg yolks (beaten)
    4 egg whites
    12 tablespoons fructose
    1 1/4 cups plus 2 tablespoons canned Pumpkin
    1/4 teaspoon Salt Sense OR pinch of Sea Salt
    1/2 teaspoon cinnamon
    1/2 teaspoon nutmeg
    1/2 teaspoon pure Vanilla Extract (no alcohol)
    Dash of allspice

Stir gelatin into cold water and dissolve rapidly. Set aside. In a double boiler cook egg yolks, 6 tablespoons fructose, pumpkin and all of the spices except the Vanilla. Stir (10-15 minutes) until thick. Remove from heat. Mix in gelatin until well blended. Refrigerate for 30 minutes until mixture begins to set. When mixture begins to set, mix in Vanilla adding 6 more tablespoons of fructose. Beat 4 egg whites until stiff. Gently fold egg whites into pumpkin mixture. Fill pie crust with mixture. Chill to set. Serve plain.

IDEA: Lite Allergy Pumpkin Pie is best eaten within 2 days.
            Make small individual pumpkin tarts.
            Layer pumpkin in a parfait glass.
IF: Use whipped cream on top of the pie garnishing with chocolate shavings.

CHAPTER 6

APPLE ENVELOPE
FILLING: 1 1/4 pounds large Golden Delicious and/or Rome Apples
2 1/2 tablespoon butter (no color added)
Optional: 2-3 tablespoons fructose

Peel and core all apples. Slice apples thin with the food processor slicing disk. Spread the apples on the pastry all but 1 1/2 inches from the edge of the dough. Fold this edge over the apples. Sprinkle with fructose and dot with butter (optional). Moisten folded edges with water. Place the top dough on. Press edges to ensure a tight fit. Make slits and holes for steam to escape. (You may need to chill extra dough in the freezer for cutting designs.) Bake in a preheated 400 degree oven 40-45 minutes until crisp. Serve warm.

DOUGH: 2 cups all purpose flour
1 1/2 sticks cold butter
1/2 cup ice water
1/8 teaspoon sea salt
Optional: 2 teaspoons fructose

In a food processor add flour and dry ingredients. Process in quick bursts 3 times. Cut butter into small pieces and add all at once. Process 5 times in short quick pulses. Do not blend butter. Add water and mix until dough just holds together 10-15 seconds. Divide dough in half. Roll out each half between 2 pieces of wax paper. Place on a cookie sheet. Let the dough rest for 30 minutes in the refrigerator.

IF: Brush pastry with egg wash (1 small egg with 1 tablespoon water) instead of water for more color when browning.

CHAPTER 6

ALLERGY ANGEL FOOD CAKE
    1 cup all purpose flour OR cake flour
    10 egg whites (use large eggs)
    1 1/4 cups fructose
    1 teaspoon cream of tartar
    1 1/2 teaspoon Vanilla Extract (no alcohol)
    1/4 teaspoon Salt Sense

    Sift or whisk flour and fructose together. Set aside. Beat egg whites with electric mixer, adding salt with cream of tartar, beating until eggs peak softly. Add vanilla at this time.
    Fold 2 tablespoons of the dry mixture into beaten egg whites <u>very gently</u> with spatula. Try to fold evenly. Dry dust a bundt pan with flour. Spoon cake mixture into the bundt pan. Bake in a preheated 325 degree oven for 45-50 minutes. Let cake cool 15 minutes before removing from pan.
Cool cake completely before frosting.

IDEA: Dribble heated Ultra Smooth Fruit Sauce over top.
           Line a jelly roll pan with wax paper(10 X 15").
           Pour batter and cook in a preheated 325 degree oven for 20 minutes. Cool 10 minutes. Fill with your favorite filling and roll up into a log cake.
IF: Dust top with powdered sugar.
           Frost with your favorite icing.

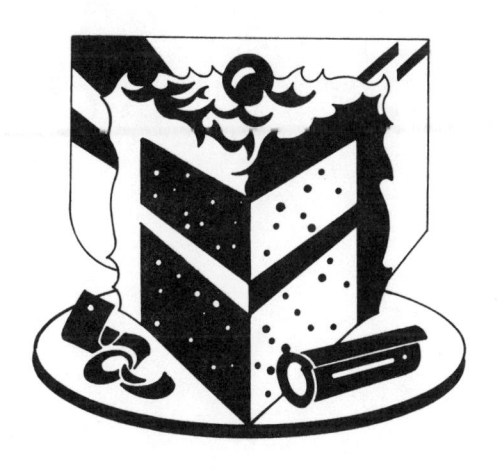

BUT I CAN'T EAT THAT

CHAPTER 6

CUSTOMIZED GRANOLA
    1/4 cup Safflower oil
    1/4 cup fructose reduced syrup*
    1 teaspoon cinnamon
    1/2 teaspoon Vanilla Extract (no alcohol)
    6 cups rolled oats (not instant)
    1 pinch sea salt
    Optional: 1/2 cup chopped dried fruits.
                  3/4 cup homemade Applesauce plain OR
                  sweetened with fructose.
                  [IF: 1/2 cup chopped nuts (almonds)]

    Preheat oven to 300-325 degrees. Mix oil with syrup adding rest of the ingredients and blend. Great eating just plain but can add extra options now. Spread thinly, on a T-FAL cookie sheet. Bake until granola is browned 20-25 minutes. For a crispier taste, stir and bake 5 minutes longer. Cool thoroughly. Keep Customized Granola in a dark cool place OR refrigerate.

*FRUCTOSE REDUCED SYRUP
    1/2 cup fructose
    1/4 cup water

    Dissolve fructose with water. In a small sauce pan whisk water mixture continuously on medium to medium high heat. Stir until mixture becomes syrupy and thick, reaching the ball stage. (As in candy making, test a drop in cold water. If it forms a ball, it is ready.)

CHAPTER 6

ALLERGY PINEAPPLE PUDDING
Serve this the same day you make it.
>1 can (20 ounce) crushed pineapple in its own juice
>1 1/2 tablespoons Arrowroot
>dash of ground cinnamon
>1 sliced banana (Optional)

Measure 1 cup of drained pineapple and set aside. In a blender, puree the rest of the pineapple with its juice until smooth. Blend Arrowroot in next. Cook in a small sauce pan over medium heat. Whisk constantly until pudding thickens. Do not boil. Remove from heat, add reserved pineapples and bananas. Spoon into parfait glasses. Chill. Sprinkle the top with cinnamon before serving.

IF: Serve with whipped cream on top.

LITE WATERMELON FREEZE
>2 quarts cut watermelon cubes, rind and seeds removed
>1/4–1/2 cup fructose

Sprinkle fruit with fructose. Freeze 5 or more hours. In the food processor puree 2 cups of frozen watermelon at a time. Mixture should be fluffy. Serve like ice cream using a scooper. This will keep frozen for 2 weeks. A notable (make ahead) lite dessert!

CHAPTER 6

ULTRA SMOOTH FRUIT SAUCE
   1 package frozen dark sweet cherries (pitted)
   1 teaspoon Arrowroot

   Defrost cherries. Pour in a small T-FAL sauce pan with a lid. Bring to a boil then reduce heat to low. Cover and simmer for 2-3 hours, occasionally mashing cherries while stirring. Cook the last 30-45 minutes uncovered to condense. Pour into a <u>blender</u> while hot. Puree smooth. Add 1 teaspoon of Arrowroot while the motor is running. This will instantly thicken. Blend 1/2 minute more. Let mixture set with the cover on the blender for 30 minutes to cool.
   Refrigerate in an air tight container. This Ultra Smooth Fruit Sauce keeps well, but does not freeze well. Use hot or cold.

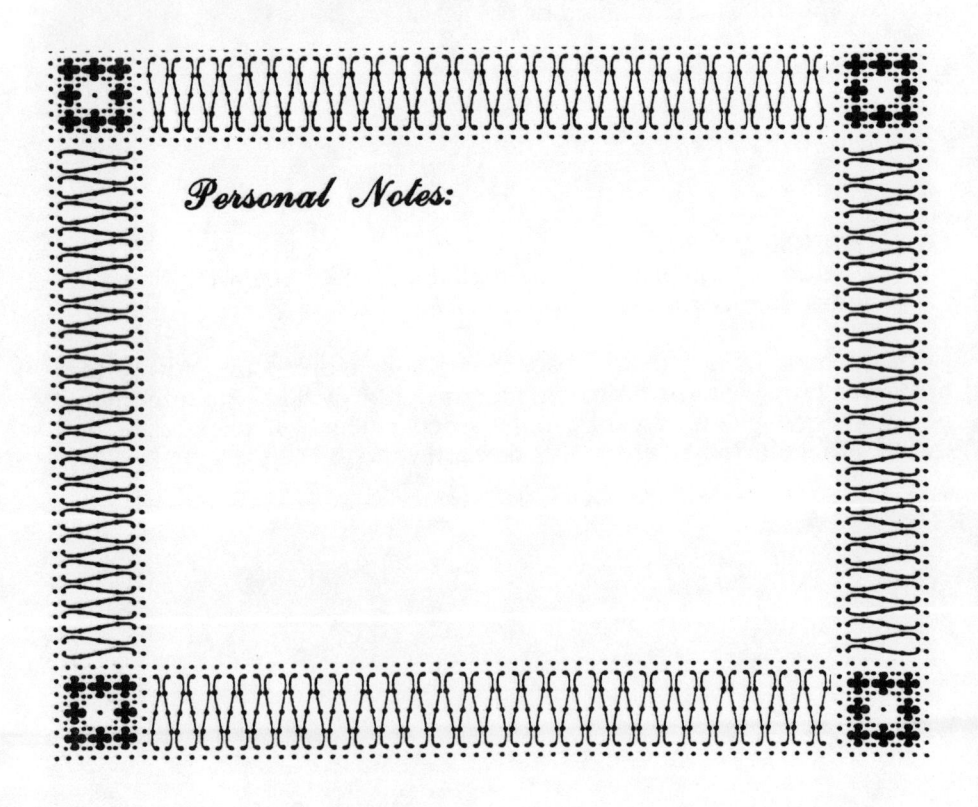

Personal Notes:

BUT I CAN'T EAT THAT

CHAPTER 6

BREAKFAST APPLE FRITTERS
    1 cup flour
    1 1/4 teaspoon homemade baking powder
    (Sift: 2 teaspoons cream of tartar, 2 teaspoons
    Arrowroot, 1 teaspoon baking soda. Measure
    given amount.)
    1/2 teaspoon Salt Sense
    1/2 teaspoon cinnamon OR nutmeg
    2 eggs
    6 tablespoons natural apple juice
    1-2 tablespoons fructose
    1 teaspoon butter OR Safflower oil
    1 cup finely chopped apples
    Safflower oil OR lard for frying

Sift or whisk dry ingredients together and set aside. Whisk wet ingredients together. Whisk dry and wet ingredients together. When the batter is ultra smooth add in the apple pieces. Drop 1 tablespoon of mixture at a time into the hot oil (375 degrees). Fry until browned on all sides. Drain and serve warm.

IF: Substitute pineapples for apples.
       Dust fritters with powdered sugar.
       Use milk instead of juice.

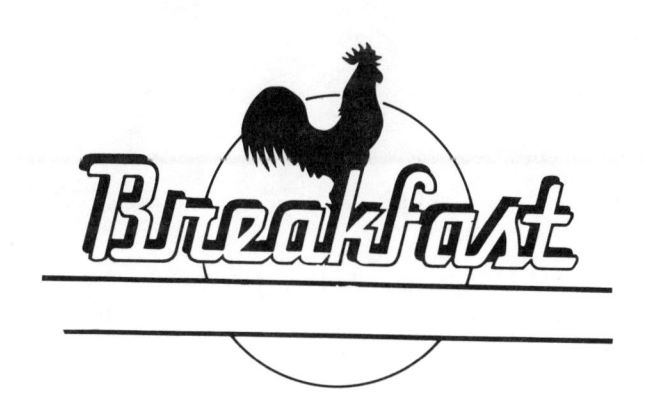

Breakfast

CHAPTER 6

ALLERGY PIZZELLES
>   2 eggs
>   6 tablespoons fructose
>   1/4 cup Safflower oil
>   2 teaspoon Vanilla Extract (no alcohol)
>   1 cup all purpose flour

Beat all ingredients together, except flour, with an electric mixer until smooth. Slowly add in the flour. Mix until smooth.

Coat the pizzelle iron with Safflower oil. Heat up the iron. Cook 1 teaspoon of batter per cookie on iron at a time, following iron's cooking instructions for the time.

IF: Use Anise, Lemon OR Almond Extracts.
        Add 1 tablespoon carob powder to the batter.

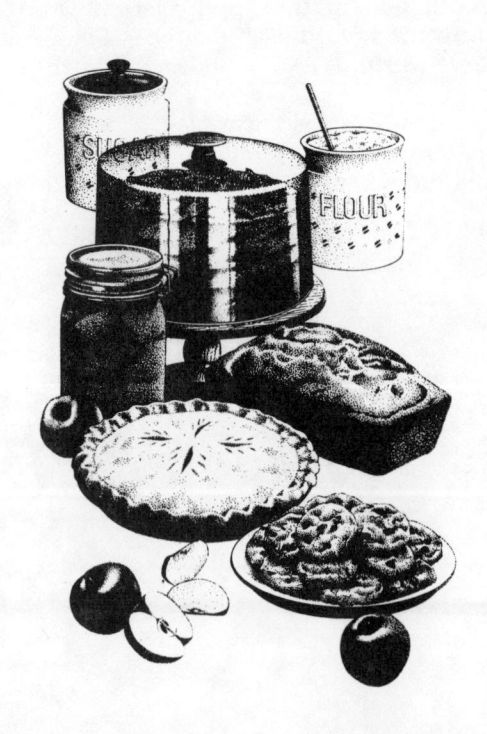

CHAPTER 6

<u>CRISP RICE TREATS</u>
    1/2 cup fructose
    1/4 cup water
    1/2 cup homemade Peanut Butter (no sugar)
    2 cup Ener-G-Crisp Rice Cereal

In a small sauce pan dissolve fructose in water. Whisk continuously on medium to medium-high heat. Stir until mixture becomes thick and syrupy, reaching the ball stage. (As in candy making, test a drop in cold water. If it forms a ball, it is ready.)

Remove from heat. Stir in peanut butter, then add in the Rice Cereal. Press into a buttered 8X8 inch pan. Cut into squares while warm. Chill in the refrigerator.

This is very sweet and you may need to cut very small pieces to control your sugar reaction. (But one is better than none!)
Crisp Rice Treats can be doubled and frozen up to 6 months.

IDEA: If you can tolerate Carob; melt carob chips with 1/2 tablespoon of unsalted butter. Thinly coat top layer before cutting. Luscious!
IF: Substitute Rice Krispies (but they do contain malt).

CHAPTER 6

BUTTERFLIES
    3 egg yolks, beaten
    1/2 teaspoon Salt Sense
    1 tablespoon fructose
    1/2 teaspoon Vanilla Extract (no alcohol)
    1/2 cup flour
    Lard for frying

    Flour a work board. Pour the flour onto the board and make a well in the middle. Add the rest of the ingredients into the well in the flour. Mix together to form a dough. Knead into a stiff dough which takes 10 minutes. Roll the dough thin and cut into 2X3 inch strips. Slash 3 slits horizontally and turn inside out and twist by putting one end through the center slit. This will look like bow ties or butterflies. Heat the oil in a skillet. Fry both sides until light brown. Makes 15 cookies.

IF: Sprinkle with powder sugar.
            Substitute 1/2 teaspoon rum OR other liqueur for vanilla. (orange, coffee, etc.)

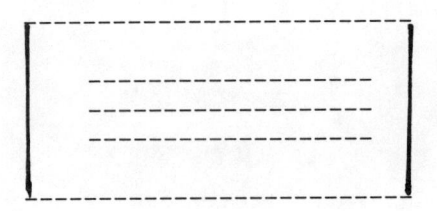

CHAPTER 6

BUTTER COOKIES

    1/2 pound real butter, room temperature (no color)
    1/2 cup fructose
    pinch of sea salt
    1/2 teaspoon Vanilla Extract (no alcohol)
    2 cup flour
    2 egg yolks

In a food processor, soften butter for 15 seconds. Add fructose, salt and vanilla, processing for 10 seconds. Add egg yolks and process 5 seconds. Add flour at one time and process 5 short pulses.

Place the dough in plastic wrap and form a log. Refrigerate overnight.

The next day slice the log into 1/2 inch rounds. Cook in a preheated 400 degree oven for 7-8 minutes. Cookies will be light in color. These cookies freeze well. Makes 4 dozen.

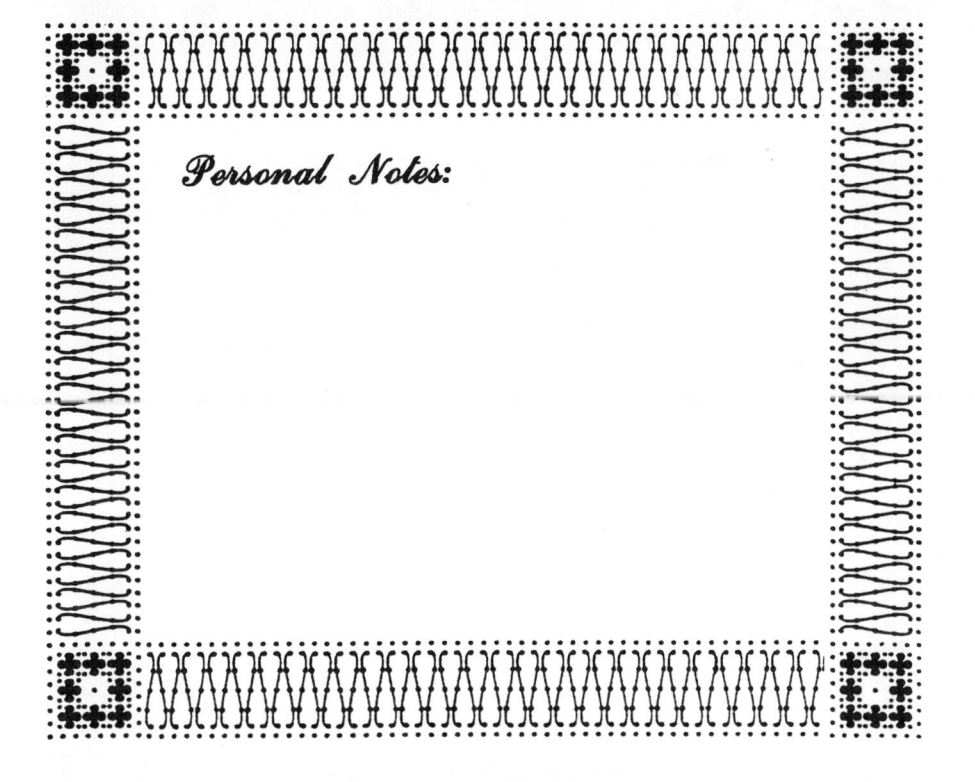

Personal Notes:

BUT I CAN'T EAT THAT

CHAPTER 6

EATABLE SHORT BREAD
    1 cup real butter (no color or additives)
    6 tablespoons fructose
    1/2 teaspoon each cinnamon, nutmeg and ginger
    dash of allspice
    2 cups all purpose flour
    1/4 teaspoon homemade baking powder
    (sift: 2 teaspoons cream of tartar, 2 teaspoons Arrowroot and
    1 teaspoon baking soda. Measure given amount.)

    Add all ingredients except butter to a food processor. Quick shift three times. Cut butter into eight pieces and add to processor while motor is running. Blend 10-15 seconds turning flour mixture into a crumbly dough. Roll dough out 1/4 inch thick on a T-Fal cookie sheet.(You can line the cookie sheet with parchment paper to prevent the bottom from burning.)
    Precut squares OR pie shapes before cooking. Prick shortbread with a tooth pick. Bake in a preheated 350 oven for 20 minutes. Cookies should be lightly browned. Recut while hot. Cool in the same pan. Makes two dozen cookies.

IDEA: <u>Cookies</u>
          Shape dough into small balls, 1 inch thick. Place on T-Fal
          cookie sheet. Press with a floured fork, stamp or glass.
          Bake in a preheated 350 degree oven for 12-15 minutes.
          Edges should be lightly browned. Makes 24 cookies
          depending on size of the cookies. Cool on a wire rack.
IF: Place jam, a nut OR a raisin in the middle of the cookies
          before baking.

Chapter 7

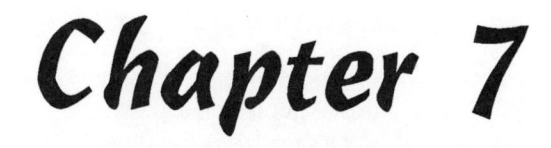

Company's Coming

Recipes for people with NO Allergies

BUT I CAN'T EAT THAT

CHAPTER 7

DIPS
Cut vegetables are grand to serve as appetizers, either plain and with dips. Your company without allergies can eat the veggies with the dips, while (you with the allergies) can eat the veggies plain with no dip. (Here's a compromise for you both without the work of making two different dishes). Prepare and cut carrots, florets of cauliflower, broccoli, sliced zucchini, celery, green or red peppers and other favorite dipping vegetables.

VEGETABLE DIP-DILL

Double	Medium	Small	batches
2	1 1/3	2/3	cups Hellman's mayo
2	1 1/3	2/3	cups sour cream
3	2	1	tablespoon dried onion
3	2	1	tablespoon dried parsley
3	2	1	teaspoon Lawry's Season Salt
3	2	1	teaspoon dillweed
1/12	1	1/2	teaspoon MSG (Accent)
1 1/2	1	1/2	Worcestershire sauce
6	4	2	drops of Tabasco sauce

Whisk all ingredients together then chill. Prepare one night before using, stirring occasionally and especially before serving. This Vegetable Dill Dip is also sensational over for baked potatoes!

VEGETABLE DIP-CURRY
  1 pint Hellman's mayo
  1/4 teaspoon dried onions
  3/4 teaspoon Worcestershire sauce
  8 drops Tabasco sauce (OR to taste)
  1/2 teaspoon curry powder
  1/2 teaspoon dried mustard
  salt and pepper to taste

Whisk all ingredients together one day before serving. Chill, stirring occasionally and especially before serving.

BUT I CAN'T EAT THAT

CHAPTER 7
APPETIZER

KAY'S CHEESE BALL
1 large package Philadelphia Cream Cheese
1 can Underwood Deviled Chicken Spread
garlic salt to taste
1/4 cup frozen chives (OR fresh)
dried parsley flakes

Bring cheese to room temperature then mix with rest of the ingredients except the parsley flakes. Shape mixture into one large ball and roll in parsley flakes until completely covered and green. Refrigerate when not using. Serve at room temperature. This cheese ball is good when made the same day needed (and for several days later but the green gets a little flattened). Serve with crackers and a spreading knife. Do not freeze.

MARIANNE'S CHICKEN DRUMETTS

Double	Single	Batches
6	3	dozen chicken drummetts (OR wings) cocktail size
2	1	cup honey
1	1/2	cup soy sauce
4	2	tablespoons oil
4	2	tablespoons ketchup
2	1	garlic clove, chopped (can use garlic powder)
2	1	13x9 inch pan

Boil all ingredients except chicken parts, until sauce thickens. Place the chicken inside a deep broiler pan(s), pour hot sauce over top of the chicken parts. Cook in a preheated 375 degree oven, basting occasionally. Bake for 75 minutes. Keep drummetts warm in a chaffing dish for the guests. This is a little on the messy side, so provide tons of napkins and your guests will love this dish.

CHAPTER 7

PEPPERONI PIZZA BREAD
    1 frozen bread dough
    1 package pepperoni slices
    1 small package shredded mozzarella cheese
    2-3 tablespoons tomato sauce

    Defrost bread at room temperature. Knead a couple of times to loosen up the gluten. Form into a square 1/4-1/2 inch thick. Spread tomato sauce over the surface and fill the center evenly with pepperoni and cheese. Roll up bread to look like a loaf. Put the seam side down on greased cookie sheet. Bake per instructions on the bread label. Slice and serve flat like pinwheels on a plate.

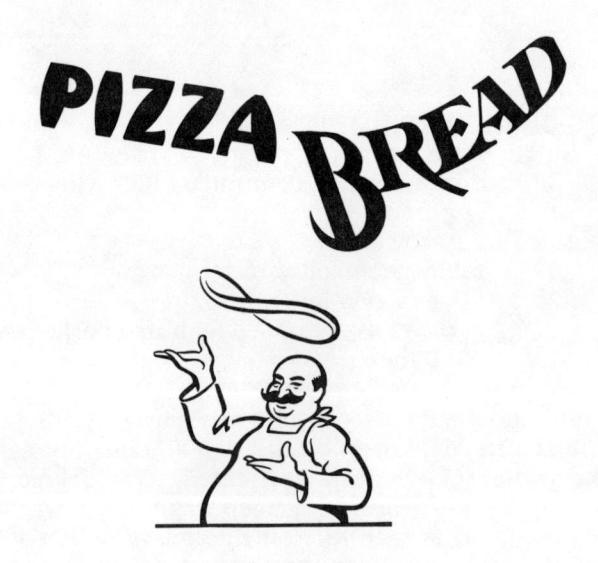

CHAPTER 7

Soup

SPLIT PEA SOUP

    1 package (16 oz.) split green peas
    2 stalks celery
    1 large carrot
    1-2 tablespoons onion powder
    1/2 teaspoon sea salt
    1 teaspoon celery salt
    1/2 teaspoon sweet basil
    2 bay leaves
    1 quart water OR Chicken Stock
    bones: beef, pork, veal OR chicken

Rinse peas several times. Soak peas overnight in plenty of hot water. Drain water in the morning. (It's surprising how much the peas do soak up.) Rinse the peas again with clear water. Add peas to stock pot with liquid and rest of the ingredients and bring to a boil. Skim the foam off from the top, cover and simmer over low heat for 2-3 hours until the peas are soft. Remove all bones and bay leaves. Discard unless you wish to use the meat from the bones in the soup. Pour the soup mixture into a Foley Food Mill and puree smooth. (A food processor will not do this correctly.) Serve with mint leaves as a garnish. Freeze excess Split Pea Soup for a nice snack on a cold winter day.

IF: For a rich, creamy soup, add 1 cup of fresh cream to the cooked soup. Reheat and serve with a tad of butter on top.

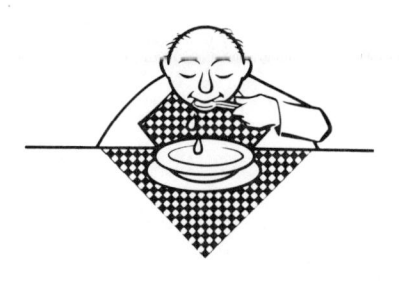

BUT I CAN'T EAT THAT

CHAPTER 7

BEEF

PLAIN GOOD BEEF STEW
    2–3 pounds of good beef stew meat (from the Butchers)
    6 carrots
    4 medium potatoes
    1 tablespoon onion powder OR 1 small onion
    OR a couple of scallions
    2 cans Cream of Mushroom Soup OR
    2 cans Cream of Celery Soup
    1 cup of gingerale
    Safflower oil

Prepare and cut vegetables. (IF: using real onions brown them first.) Mix all ingredients together. Put mixture into the Dutch Oven and cook in a preheated 300 degree oven for 3 hours. Stir occasionally. Meat will brown and gravy will thicken automatically. You can add 1/2 cups of bread crumbs over top for the last half hour.

SHARON'S COMPANY CASSEROLE

Double	Single	recipes
2	1	pound ground beef sirloin
whole	1/2	package noodles (thinner noodles)
1	1/2	teaspoon seasoned salt
2	1	can(s) tomato sauce
1	1/2	cup cottage cheese
1	1/2	tablespoon onion salt
1	1/2	pound shredded Cheddar cheese

Cook noodles according to instructions on package <u>but cook 4 minutes less</u>. Brown meat and drain. Mix tomato sauce in and simmer. Mix in drained noodles with the rest of the ingredients and place into a large casserole dish. Bake uncovered in a preheated 350 degree oven for 30 minutes. Large recipe serves 10 people. Small recipe serves 5 people.

CHAPTER 7

ROYAL CHICKEN
  6-7 Chicken breasts (skins on OR off)
  1/2 cup of clarified butter OR margarine
  (The milk solids in the butter will burn)
  1/2 cup bread crumbs
  1/2 cup grated cheese (Parmesan sticks best)
  1 1/2 tablespoons parsley flakes
  garlic salt and onion powder to taste
  ground black pepper (optional)

Mix crumbs together with spices and cheese. Dip chicken into the melted butter then coat with bread crumbs. (I put them all together in a plastic bag and just shake.) Place chicken in a 13 x 9 inch pan bone side up, meat side down. Dribble the rest of the butter over the top of the chicken. Do not turn chicken while cooking. Bake in a preheated 350 degree oven for 65-70 minutes, (depending how big the breasts are). The meat stays tender and has a very crispy crust. This is great for company!

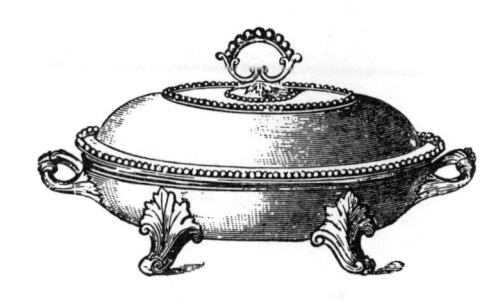

BUT I CAN'T EAT THAT

CHAPTER 7

EGGS

SWEET AND SOUR EGGS
    4 eggs
    1 teaspoon water (times 4)
    1/2 cup plus 1 tablespoon Chicken Stock
    1 tablespoon peanut oil
    2 tablespoons sugar
    2 tablespoons white vinegar
    1 teaspoon tomato paste OR ketchup
    1/2 teaspoon salt
    1 tablespoon cornstarch
    4 water chestnuts, cut thin
    1 carrot, cut in small wedges
    1 clove garlic OR garlic powder

    Mix together stock, garlic, oil, sugar, vinegar, paste, salt and cornstarch, stirring constantly. Bring mixture to a boil. Add sliced water chestnuts and carrots. Simmer for 5 minutes.
    Beat each egg separately with 1 teaspoon of water in each egg, making 4 individual omelets. Fold omelets when cooked in half and in half again. Arrange two egg triangles slightly on top of each other and pour Sweet and Sour Sauce over tops. Serve hot. Serves 2 people. This is an excellent recipe for a romantic breakfast.

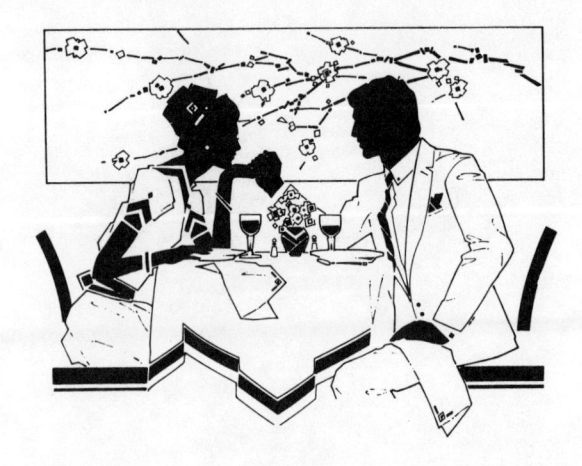

CHAPTER 7

SANDRA'S TWO CHEESE STRATA

Double	Single	Recipes
8	4	large eggs, beaten
10	5	slices of bread
1 1/2	1 cup	shredded colby OR mild longhorn cheese
1 1/2	1 cup	shredded muenster OR mozzarella cheese
2 1/2	1 1/4	cup Half and Half cream
1/2	1/4	teaspoon seasoned salt
1/2	1/4	teaspoon dry mustard
1/4	1/8	teaspoon nutmeg
1	1/2	stick of butter at room temperature

Optional:

    For **MEAT STRATA** use cooked Canadian Bacon, cooked sausage OR cooked ground meat.

    For **VEGETABLE STRATA** use a sliced zucchini, 1 sliced red pepper, 1/4 cup parsley, 1/2 teaspoon oregano, 1 teaspoon sweet basil and 1/2 teaspoon onion powder.

    Cut the crusts off of bread slices. Butter both sides of bread and cut into fourths. Grease a 9 x 13 inch pan. Line half of the bread on the bottom. Layer with half amount of cheeses. Add another layer of remaining bread over top of cheese layer, then add the remaining cheese. (Top with meat OR sliced vegetables OR place them in middle of a layer.) Mix the remaining ingredients together and pour over the top. Cover and refrigerate over night. Bring to room temperature before cooking. Bake uncovered for 45 minutes to 1 hour in a preheated 325-350 degree oven. Strata should be firm and browned on top. Let it stand 10 minutes before cutting. Large recipe serves 12 to 14 people. Small recipe serves 6 to 8 people. (There are usually no leftovers, but if so, it does reheat nicely in the oven.)

CHAPTER 7

VEGGIES

CHEESE BROCCOLI CASSEROLE

Double	Single	Recipes
1	1/2	stick of butter
1	1/2	teaspoon onion powder
2	1	box (12 oz.) frozen chopped broccoli
3	1 1/2	cups cooked rice
1	1/2	can cream of chicken soup
1/2	1/2	cup of milk
1 cup (8 oz.)	1/2 cup (4 oz.)	– Cheese Whiz

                                  Red peppers for garnish
                                  mushrooms (optional)

Sauté onion powder and broccoli in butter. Mix in the rest of the ingredients. Pour into a greased casserole dish. Bake uncovered in a preheated 350 degree oven for 30 minutes. Garnish with 3 red pepper rings after cooked. This is a great dish reheated if there's any left over.

BROCCOLI MARINADE

    1 bunch fresh broccoli
    6 tablespoons Safflower oil mixed with:
        1/4 teaspoon dry mustard
        3/4 teaspoon salt
        dash of pepper
        2 tablespoons cider vinegar
    Topping:
        3/4 cup Hellman's mayo thinned with 3 tablespoons of fresh lemon juice

Wash and clean broccoli. Cut stalks in half lengthwise for long bushy pieces. Blanch in boiling hot water until stalks are bright green, 1-3 minutes, then dip immediately in ice cold water to stop the cooking action. Drain broccoli. Marinate in oil mixture overnight turning when possible. A plastic bag makes this procedure easy. The next day drain. Fan broccoli out on a serving plate and pour topping over the top to jazz it up. Serve as a cold side dish.

IDEA: Use raw broccoli and the topping as dip.

CHAPTER 7

JELLO

FAMILY'S FAVORITE JELLO

Double	Single	recipes
1	1/2	large package Royal Cherry Gelatin (OR Jell-O)
1	1/2	cup sour cream
1	1/2	cup large can cranberry jelly

Make Jello according to directions, minus 1/2 cup of liquid for a double batch, OR minus 1/4 cup of liquid for a single batch. Refrigerate Jello until semi set, 1/2-1 hour. In a blender mix sour cream with cranberry jelly (food processor doesn't work as well in blending.) Add this mixture with the semi set Jello also in the blender. Pour into a wet mold. Refrigerate until firm. Invert mold pan and slip onto a serving plate.

LIME SUPREME (JELL-O)
1 small package Royal Lime Gelatin
(or Jell-O)
1/2 cup hot water
1 can (8 oz) Bartlett pears in its own juice
1 package Dream Whip (OR Cool Whip)
1 pkg.(3 oz.) Philadelphia cream cheese (at room temperature)

Melt Jello in hot water. In a blender add Jello and cream cheese. Blend until smooth. Add canned pears with juice to the blender mixture. Blend until smooth.

Mix Dream Whip per directions. Lightly fold Dream Whip into pear mixture. Pour into a wet mold and refrigerate until firm. Invert mold pan and slip onto a serving plate.

CHAPTER 7

GREAT PIE CRUST

    4 cups all purpose flour
    1 tablespoon sugar
    1 teaspoon salt
    1 3/4 cups solid Crisco shortening
    1/2 cup cold water
    1 tablespoon lemon juice
    1 large egg

Whisk all dry ingredients together. Make a well in the center of the bowl. In another bowl whisk all of the wet ingredients together, except shortening. Using a pastry cutter (OR two knives), cut shortening into the dry ingredients until dough looks crumbly and resembles the size of small peas. Moisten this with the wet mixture using a fork with a light touch. Divide dough into four portions. Wrap each portion in plastic and refrigerate for 1/2 hour or more. Roll out when chilled between two sheets of wax paper. Place dough in pie pan and prick. Line the top of the pie crust with foil and fill with beans for weight. Cook in a preheated 450 degree oven for 10 minutes for a single cooked pie crust to be filled as you wish.

IDEAS: To make pie crust richer tasting use half Crisco and half butter in recipe. It is handy to have an extra sheet of pie crust on hand. Roll out dough and freeze flat, to be ready when needed.

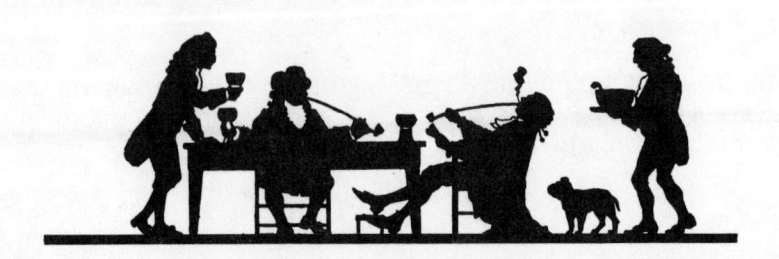

CHAPTER 7

DESERTS

MOTHERS-IN-LAW'S COFFEE CAKE (Breakfast)
Your mother-in-law will love this!
>1/4 pound of butter (at room temperature)
>1 cup sugar
>3 eggs
>2 cups flour
>1 teaspoon baking powder
>1 teaspoon baking soda
>1/4 teaspoon salt
>1 cup sour cream

Topping:
>1 3/4 cup brown sugar
>2 tablespoons flour
>2 teaspoons cinnamon
>4-5 tablespoons of butter
>1 cup chopped, minced OR chunky pecans (optional)

With an electric mixer, cream together the butter and sugar. Add in one egg at a time beating well with each addition. Whisk all of the dry ingredients together to sift. Add to cream mixture alternating with sour cream, adding a little at a time. Batter will be thick. Spread in a buttered 13x9x2 inch baking dish. Mix topping in the food processor to evenly cut in butter. Sprinkle topping over the top of the cake mixture. Dot with more butter. Bake in a preheated 325-350 oven for 30-40 minutes until done. Cut into squares. Serving hot or cold.

CHAPTER 7

CREAM CHEESE CAKE

1/4 pound butter
1 1/2 cups (14 crackers) Cinnamon Crisp Graham Crackers
(if using plain graham crackers add 1/4 cup powdered sugar plus
1 teaspoon cinnamon)
1 (8 oz.) Philadelphia Cream Cheese
2 egg yolks
1/2 teaspoon Vanilla Extract
pinch of salt
6 tablespoons milk OR cream (1/3 cup)
2 tablespoons flour
1/3 cup sugar
2 egg whites

Topping:
1/2 pint sour cream
3 tablespoons sugar
1/2 teaspoon Vanilla Extract

Garnish:
Use crushed graham crackers, melted blueberry sauce
OR chocolate shavings.

In the microwave, soften cream cheese for 30 seconds on 50% power. Set aside. Microwave butter for 75 seconds on 70% power. Crush graham crackers in the food processor. Mix melted butter with the crackers and press into a 9 inch cake pan. Press firmly into the pan using the back of a large spoon.

Mix the cream cheese with 2 egg yolks, vanilla, salt and beat well with the electric mixer. Add milk, flour and sugar to mixture while beating. In a separate bowl beat the egg whites until stiff. Gently fold the beaten egg whites into the cheese mixture. Pour all into the graham cracker crust. Bake in a preheated 325 degree oven for 35-45 minutes. Remove from oven.

Turn the oven up to 400 degrees. Mix up topping and pour over the top of the cooked cheese cake. Bake 5 more minutes.

Garnish with crumbs, drizzle warm blueberry sauce over top, swirl melted chocolate OR shave chocolate over the top of cheese cake.

CHAPTER 7

BOSTON CREAM PIE

This Boston Cream Pie is really a cake! Here's a quick and easy way to make this great dessert!

Bake one recipe of your favorite yellow cake from scratch. (Or use a mix.) Cool and cut in half, splitting the layers horizontally using the string method. Make as many layers as you wish

Mix up a batch of your favorite vanilla pudding from scratch. (OR use a mix.) Fill the layer in between the cakes with pudding. Place top of cake back on top of last pudding layer.
NOW THIS IS THE FUN PART!

The Chocolate Glaze

1. Melt in the microwave 3 tablespoons butter and 3 squares (1 oz. each) unsweetened chocolate, stir a couple of times watching carefully.

2. Stir in 1 cup of powdered sugar, 3/4 teaspoon Vanilla Extract and 1-2 tablespoons hot water to get the desired consistency of a glaze.

3. Pour the Chocolate Glaze over the top of the cake letting it run over the sides in streams. <u>You must work fast</u>!! Chill until needed. Serve Boston Cream Pie the same day you make it. Keeps only one day in the refrigerator.

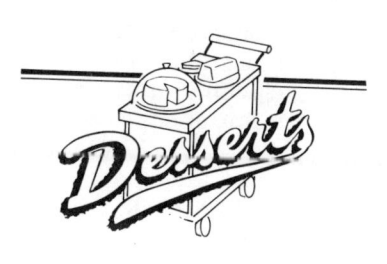

CHAPTER 7

POTATO CHIP COOKIES
1 cup minus 2 tablespoons unsalted butter
1 1/4 cup flour
1/2 cup sugar
1 cup crushed potato chips
1 teaspoon Vanilla Extract
(optional):
1/2 cup crushed nuts (reduce chips to 1/2 cup chips when using nuts)

Mix ingredients together in the order given. Drop 1 full teaspoon of cookie dough on a T-Fal cookie sheet. Bake preheated 350 degree oven for 15-20 minutes. Cookies brown quickly so you might want to use a sheet of parchment paper underneath. Dust powdered sugar over top of cookies, when cool.

WALNUT BARS
1/2 stick butter
2 cups brown sugar
3 eggs beaten
2 cups flour
2 teaspoons baking powder
pinch of salt
1 teaspoon Vanilla Extract
1 cup fine chopped walnuts (OR pecans)

Butter and flour a 9x13x2 inch pan. Mix all ingredients together in order. Add batter to the pan and smooth the top with a spatula. Bake in a preheated 350 degree oven for 30-35 minutes. Sprinkle with powdered sugar when hot and again when serving. Cut cake into long finger bars. Bars keep very well.

CHAPTER 7

FUDGE MELT AWAY'S
Layer #1
- 1/2 cup butter
- 1 square of unsweetened chocolate
- 1/2 cup granulated sugar
- 1 teaspoon Vanilla Extract
- 1 cup shredded coconut
- 1/2 cup chopped nuts
- 1 beaten egg
- 2 cups of crushed Honey Graham Crackers

Melt butter with chocolate carefully in the microwave. Mix in sugar, vanilla, shredded coconut, chopped nuts, egg and crushed Honey Graham Crackers. Press this into an ungreased 11x7 inch pan. Cool in the refrigerator until firm 1-1 1/2 hours.

Layer #2
- 1/4 cup butter
- 2 tablespoons cream OR milk
- 1 teaspoon Vanilla Extract
- 2 cups powdered sugar

Melt butter in the microwave. Mix cream, vanilla and powdered sugar into the melted butter. Pour this over the first layer quickly and evenly. Cool 1/2 hour in refrigerator.

Layer #3
- 2 squares of unsweetened chocolate
- 2 tablespoons of butter

For the last layer melt 2 squares of unsweetened chocolate with 2 tablespoons of butter in the microwave. Pour this over the white layer #2 and refrigerate. Cut before cookies become to solid. Chill completely. Keep chilled until the last minute, they melt as fast as the disappear!

BUT I CAN'T EAT THAT

CHAPTER 7
CARROT AND PINEAPPLE CAKE
Very moist and delicious!
- 2 1/4 cups all purpose flour
- 2 teaspoons baking soda
- 2 teaspoons baking powder
- 1 teaspoon salt
- 1 tablespoon cinnamon
- 1/4 teaspoon nutmeg
- 1/4 teaspoon allspice
- 1 can (15 oz.) crushed pineapple (well drained)
- 4-5 medium carrots (shredded)
- 5 small eggs
- 1 3/4+ cups of sugar
- 1 cup Safflower Oil
- 1/2 cup melted butter
- 1 1/2 teaspoon Vanilla Extract

Process first 7 ingredients in the food processor for 4 seconds. Remove from bowl and place on waxed paper. Drain the pineapple, pressing all of the liquid out with the back of a large spoon. Discard liquid. Peel and fine shred carrots, set aside. Add eggs and sugar to processor. Blend for 1 1/2 minutes until light in color. Melt butter in the microwave for 50 seconds on high. Mix melted butter with the oil. <u>With processor running</u>, pour in the oil mixture, slowly blending it into the egg and sugar mixture for 1-2 minutes. Mixture should be fluffy. Add vanilla, carrots and pineapple, processing 2-3 quick pulses. Pour dry mixture through feeding tube turning processor on and off 4-5 times until flour is absorbed. Do not over mix. Pour into a greased and floured 12 cup bundt pan. Bake in a preheated 325/350 degree oven for 60-65 minutes until cake pulls away from the sides. Let cake cool 10 minutes before removing it from the pan to cool on a wire rack.

CREAM CHEESE FROSTING
- 1 (6 oz.) Philly Cream Cheese (room temperature)
- 4 cups powdered sugar
- 1 stick butter (room temperature)
- pinch of salt
- 1 teaspoon Vanilla Extract

In a mixer, whip cream cheese and butter until smooth. Add vanilla and salt. Gradually add powdered sugar. Mix until smooth and creamy to a good spreading consistency. Frost entire cake when cool. Refrigerate cake 5 hours OR overnight. Serve cold. This cake is very rich so I suggest serving thin slices. Carrot and Pineapple cake freezes well.

*This recipe may be made entirely with a mixer if not in possession of a food processor.

SAFE AND ACCESSIBLE FOODS

*=Health Food Store
*=probable purchase place
**=Wheat, Color (artificial), Malt, Preservatives OR Chemicals (I.E.: sulfates), Sugar (cane)

CEREALS	COMPANY	**CONTAINS No:
Apple Corns	Arrowhead Mills P.O.Box 2059 Herford, TX 79045	W C P S
*Health Food Store		
Aztec Cereal	Erewhon	W C M P S
*Health Food Store		
Corn Apple	Arrowhead Mills	W C M P S
*Health Food Store		
Corn Flakes	Arrowhead Mills	W C M P S
*Health Food Store		
Crispy Brown Rice	Perky Foods	W C M P S
*Grocery or Health Food		
Puffed Rice (Brown)	Arrowhead Mills	W C M P S
*Health Food Store		
Fruit Lites (Corn)	Healthy Valley Inc. 16100 Foothill Blvd. Irwindale, CA 91706-7811	W C M P S
Puffed Rice (White)	Malt-O-Meal	W C M P S
*Grocery		
(Cream of Brown Rice) Quick'N Creamy	Pacific Rice Products Woodland, CA 95695	W C M P S
*Health Food Store		
Cream of Brown Rice	Lundberg Farms P.O.Box 369 Richval, CA 95974	W C M P S
*Health Food Store		
(Cream of Brown Rice) Rice Bran	Hodgson P.O.Box 430 Teutopolis, IL 62467	W C M P S
*Grocery		

SAFE AND ACCESSIBLE FOODS

Cream of Buckwheat	Pocono, Heart of Buckwheat Brand	W C M P S
*Health Food Store Cream of Rye	Roman Meal Co. Tacoma, WA 98411-0126	W C M P S
*Health Food Store Rice Nuts	Ener-G-Foods 5960 1st Ave. Seattle, WA 98124-5787	W C M P S
*Health Food Store Direct from Co.		

CARBOHYDRATES

No Yeast Brown Rice *Health Food Store/ Direct from company	Ener-G Foods Variety Products	W C M P S
Scalette (Sicilian Specially Bread) *Grocery		C M P S
Rice: Short and Sweet, Wehani, Jubilee *Grocery/Health Food	Lundberg Farms Walnut Acres	W C M P S
Rice Pasta Elbows Rice Spaghetti	Pastariso 55 Ironside Crescent Units 6&7 Scarborough, Ontario, M1X1N3	W C M P S
Fruits-Natural Applesauces, Peach Sauces, etc. *Grocery	Beach-Nut Baby Foods Senaca/Motts	W C M P S
Drinks After the Fall spritzers/juices *Health Food Stores	After the Fall Walnut Acres	C M P S
Distilled water *Grocery or Direct from company	Distillata Co. Cleveland, Ohio 44114	C
Rice Lites (non-dairy drink) *Health Food Store	Imagine Foods Inc. 350 Cambridge Ave. Palo Alto, CA 94301	W C M P S

SAFE AND ACCESSIBLE FOODS
DESERTS

Brown Rice Treat	Glenny's Glenn Foods 999 Central Ave. Woodmere, N.Y. 11598	W C M P S
Rice Dream (non-dairy ice cream) *Health Food Store	Imagine Foods Inc. 350 Cambridge Ave. Palo Alto, CA 94306	W C M P S

SNACKS:

Brown Rice Chips	Amsnack Milwaukee, Wisc. 53209	W C M P S
*Health Food Store		
Charlie Chips potato chips *Grocery	Charlie Chips	C P S
Crisp Bread Rye Crackers *Grocery	WASA	W C M P S
Poppers	Natures Warehouse	W C M P
Jam filled pastry *Health Food Store	Walnut Acres	

Oils and Spices

Bob Evans Lard *Grocery	Bob Evans	C P
Breakstone Butter *Grocery	Breakstone	C P
Safflower Oil *Grocery/Health Store	Hollywood Arrowhead Mills	C P
Sea Salt *Health Food Store		P
Pure Vanilla Flavoring (no alcohol)	Spicery Shoppe Downers Grove, IL. 60515	C P S

AGENCIES AND PEOPLE TO CONTACT

Allergy Foundation of America
801 Second Ave.
New York, New York
10017
212-684-7875

Allergy Information Association
65 Tromely Drive. Suite 10
Etobicoke, Ontario
Canada, M9B5Y7

Asthma and Allergy Foundation of America
1717 Massachusetts Ave.
NW 20036
Information, referrals services and speakers; conducts programs for asthmatic children and their parents; scholarships for asthmatic athletes.
265-0265

Hyperactive Children's Support Group
c/o Sally Bunday
71 Whyke Lane
Chichester
West Sussex, England
PO192LD

National Digestive Diseases Information Clearinghouse
P.O. Box NDDIC
Bethesda, MD
20892
301-468-6344
IBS, Metabolic diseases,
Digestive and Diabetes,
Kidney

National Foundation for Allergy
(National Institutes of Health)
9000 Rockville Pike
Bethesda, MD
20892
Information 1-301-496-5717

AGENCIES AND PEOPLE TO CONTACT

National Library of Medicine
8600 Rockville Pike
Bethesda, MD
20894
Information 301-496-6308

Vitality Health Food
c/o David Vitantonio
28202 Chardon Road
Willoughby Hills, Ohio
44092
216-585-8575

Ireland Cancer Center
University Hospitals of Cleveland
2074 Abington Road
Cleveland, OH 44106
216-844-3951
Support group for cancer survivors
and families.

American Cancer Society-Headquarters
1599 Clifton Rd. N.E.
Atlanta, Georgia 30329
Public Information Programs

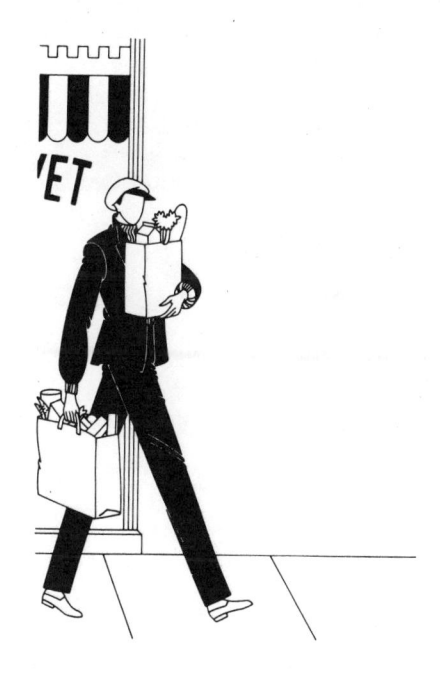

RECOMMENDED READING

Allergies (Encyclopedia of Health)
Edward Edelson
Chelsea House Publishers 1989

Allergy-Self Help Book
Sharon Faelten
Rodale Press 1983

The Asthma Self Help Book
Paul J. Hannaway MD.
Lighthouse Press 1989

Best Guide to Allergy
Giannini MD., Schultz MD.
Chang MD. and Wong
Appleton-Century-Crofts 1981

The Complete Book of Salads
Alessandra Vallone
Gallery Books

The Diet Principal
Victoria Principal
Simon and Schuster 1987

Fresh; A Green Market Cookbook
Carol Schneider
Panache Press

Help Me To Help My Child
Jill Bloom
Little, Brown and Co. 1990

Helping Your Hyperactive Child
John F. Taylor, Ph.D.
Prima Publishing and Communications
1990

The Gluten-Free Gourmet
Bette Hagman
Holt 1990

RECOMMENDED READING

How To Find Relief From Migraine
R. Dudley and W. Rowland
Beautfort Books Inc. 1982

The New Pastry Cook
Helen Fletcher
William Morrow and Co. Inc.

Relief From IBS
Elaine Fantle Shimberg
M. Evans and Co.

The Sugar Dilemma
R.Martens MD. and S.Martens MS.RD.
Medi-Ed Press 1987
(Lactose Intolerance)

The Way To Cook
Julia Child
Alfred A. Knopf 1989

Yeast Free Living
A.Annechild and L.Johnson
Putnam Publishing Group 1986
(Candidas)

Your Hyperactive Child, Adolescent and Adult
Paul Wander MD.
Oxford University Press 1987

Hypoglycemia: A Better Approach
Paavo Airola Ph.D.
Health Plus Publishers 1977

Complete Guide to Pregnancy
Columbus University College of Physicians
and Surgeons
Crown Publishers   1988

Cancer and Nutrition
Elizabeth Somer MA. RD.
Grolier Educational Corp.   1988

REFERENCES

<u>Allergy Self-Help Cook Book</u>
Marjorie Hurt Jones RN.
Rodale Press 1984
<u>American Medical Association</u>
Family Medical Guide
Random House 1987
<u>Better Homes and Garden Fresh Fish Cookbook</u>
Meredith Corporation 1989
<u>Cecil Textbook of Medicine</u>
Wyngearden and Smith
W.B. Saunders Co. 1985
<u>The Complete Family Cookbook</u>
Curtin Productions Inc. 1969
<u>Cooking A To Z</u>
Jane Horn
Otho Books 1988
<u>Cutting Up in the Kitchen</u>
Merle Ellis
Chronicle Books 1977
<u>Disease Data Book</u>
J.Fry, G.Sandler and D.Brooks
MTP Press Limited 1986
<u>Easy Cooking-32 Zesty Pizzas</u>
B.Bennett and K.Upton
Barron's 1983
<u>The Family Mental Health Encyclopedia</u>
Frank J. Bruno Ph.D.
John Wiley and Sons Publishers 1989
<u>Fabulous Fructose Recipe Book</u>
J.Cooper MD. and J.Jones.
M.Evans and Co. Inc. 1979

REFERENCES

Fannie Farmer Cookbook
Boston Cooking School Cookbook 10th Ed.
Bantam Books 1972

Food Values
J.Pennington and H.Church
Harper and Row 1985

The Herb and Spice Cookbook
Sheryl and Mel London
Rondale Press 1986

Joy of Cooking
I.Rombauer and M.Becker
Signet 1974

Menus for Pasta
Anna Tresa Callen
Crown Publishers Inc. 1985

The New Child Health Encyclopedia
Boston Children's Hospital
Delacorte Press 1987

New Double Day Cookbook
J.Anderson and E.Hanna
Double Day and Co. 1985

Nurses Reference Library Diagnostics
2nd Ed.
Springhouse Corp. 1986

Nutrition Almanac
John D. Kirschmann
McGraw-Hill Book Co. 1979

Perfect Pasta
Valentina Harris
William Morrow and Co. Inc. 1984

Principles of Nutrition and Diet Therapy
Barbara Luke
Little Brown and Co. 1984

Professional Guide to Diseases
3rd. Edition
Springhouse Corp. 1989

Statistical Abstract of U.S. 1990
U.S.Department of Commerce
Bureau of the Census 1990

Step By Step Mexican Cooking
Gallery Books 1989

Rice Dream™
NON-DAIRY DESSERT

IMAGINE FOODS, INC.

BUT I CAN'T EAT THAT

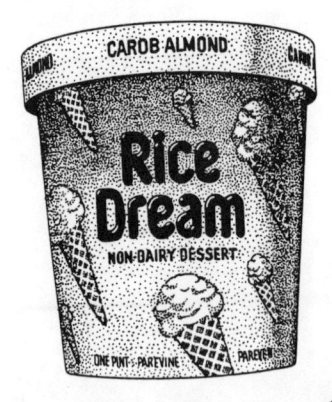

Soft Serve Rice Dream™

RICE DREAM

RICE DREAM

NON DAIRY BEVERAGE

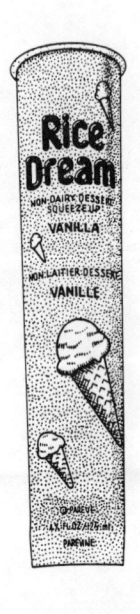

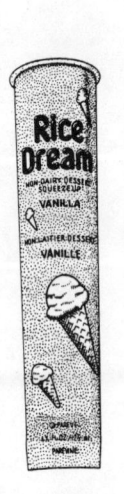

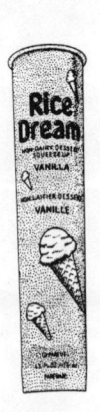

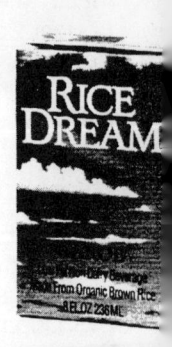

IMAGINE
FOODS

Ⓤ PAREVE

Walnut Acres
ORGANIC FARMS • SINCE 1946

Penns Creek, Pennsylvania 17862   Phone: 717-837-0603   Fax: 717-837-1146

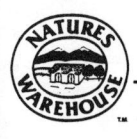

Natures Warehouse, Inc.
P.O. Box 161525, Sacramento, CA 95816

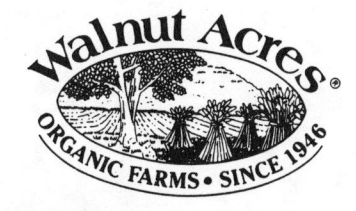

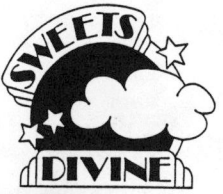

Walnut Acres
ORGANIC FARMS • SINCE 1946

Rice Syrup Sweetened
Sweets Divine Candy Bars

North Woods Rice
NET WT. 16 OZ. (1 LB.)

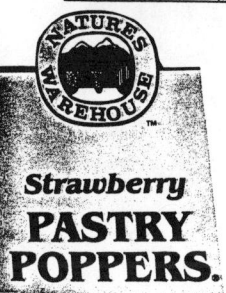

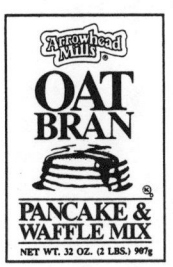

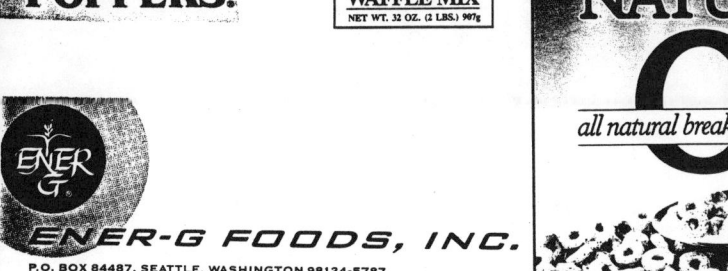

Strawberry PASTRY POPPERS

Arrowhead Mills OAT BRAN PANCAKE & WAFFLE MIX
NET WT. 32 OZ. (2 LBS.) 907g

Arrowhead Mills NATURE O's
all natural breakfast cereal
NO SALT OR SUGAR ADDED

ENER-G FOODS, INC.
P.O. BOX 84487, SEATTLE, WASHINGTON 98124-5787
Telephone 1-800-331 5222, in Washington State 1-800-325-9788

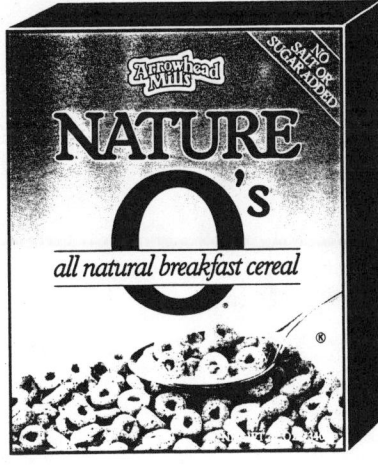

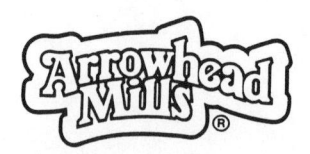

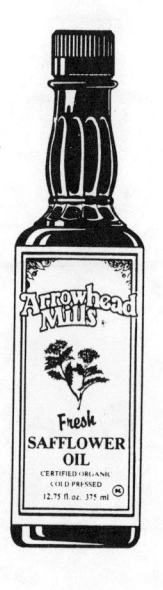

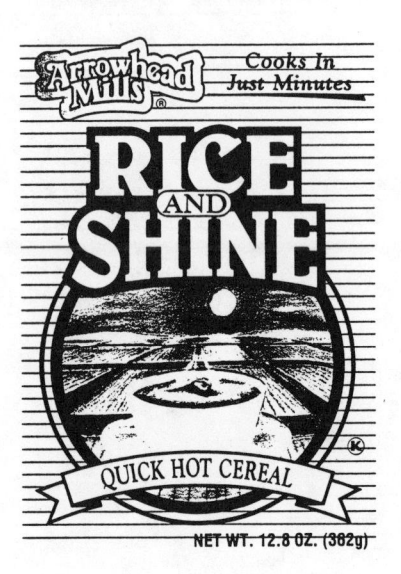

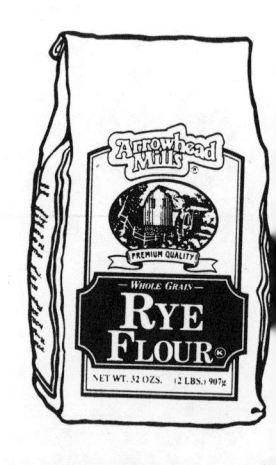

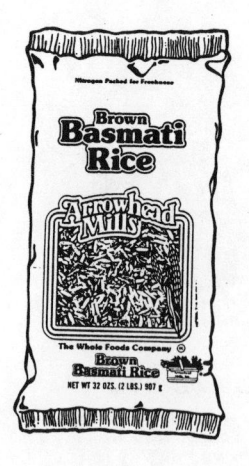

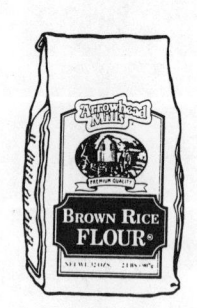

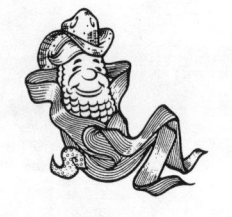

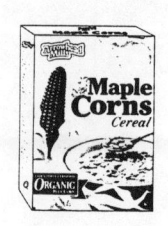

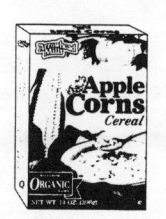

Addendum

But I Can't Eat That can benefit people with these other health problems.

Illness:

Allergies and Food Sensitivities

Hyperactivity and ADHD

Hypoglycemia and Hyperglcemia

Candidas

Stomach Ulcers

Queasy Pregnancies

Celiac Disease

IBS

Cancer

ADDENDUM

ILLNESS

Always refer to your Doctor for professional advice.
Keeping this in mind, I would like to touch lightly upon illness and/or disorders that would benefit from But I Can't Eat THAT. These are allergies, hyperactivity, food sensitivities, hypoglycemia, Candidas, Morning Sickness, stomach ulcers, IBS (intestinal problems) and eating problems connected with cancer treatments. To keep flare ups to a minimum these difficulties means maintaining a non-irritating and (sometimes) bland diet, sometimes indefinitely. Some disorders are life long with no cure. Others are just enough to disturb normal life. Both need to be addressed and taken care of to enjoy an improved life style.

Frequent meals are recommended for easier digestion and absorption. This gives the person an added advantage to maintain even blood (sugar) levels, thus giving the person a better mental out look. This is very important to succeed. The timing of these meals runs; breakfast, mid morning, lunch, mid afternoon, dinner and bed time.

Electrolytes is a safe item to have around the house at all times. This works better than water to hydrate the body. Electrolytes meet the body's requirements of potassium, phosphate, sodium, positive and negative ions to maintain the proper acid base. This balance is especially needed in illness, flu and heat sickness by preventing dehydration. A good source of electrolytes is found in water solutions by Pedilyte, Lytren Nursette and Ricelyte.

Again, let your Doctor put together a list of requirements for your specific problems. Many of the recipes in But I Can't Eat That will meet the requirements.

Allergies and food sensitivities are virtually one and the same (in my option). Allergies can be proven and sensitivities can't, but you are ill from both.

ILLNESS (Cont.)

Allergies and Food Sensitivities symptoms vary from headaches (migraines), lethargy, nausea, confusion, dermatitis (rashes and hives) to behavioral changes (mood swings, depression, hyperactivity), gastrointestinal problems (colitis) and respiratory problems (stuffiness, runny eyes, asthma). Reaction times vary from 5 minutes (immediate) to 72 hours (delayed) after being in contact with OR digesting irritants. Altering food proteins may not have the same reaction (I.E., heating OR freezing). Remember, alcohol makes the offending food penetrate faster and more intensely.

Here are items often eliminated from diets for allergies.

Yeast and Molds:	breads, cheese, dairy, dried fruits, lunch meats, malt, organ meats. Eating fresh foods within a 18 to 24 hour period ensures no molds. To store, freeze after this period. Defrost and eat immediately.
Coal Tar Products:	artificial colors, aspirin
Citric:	grapefruits, lemon, limes, oranges
Caffeine:	chocolate, coffee, coke, tea
Additives and Chemicals:	artificial colors, monosodium glutamate (MSG), preservatives, extracts, sulfates, artificial sweeteners
Hydrogenated Oils:	are found in tons of products.
Nightshade Family:	eggplant, potatoes, some squashes, tomatoes
Others:	barley, beef, broccoli, corn, cucumber, malt, onions, wheat

Hyperactivity Avoiding sugars (I.E., corn syrup, lactose, dextrose, saccharin, cane sugars) does help this situation greatly. Hyperactivity can come hand in hand with allergies and ADHD.

ADHD (Attention Deficit Hyperactivity Disorder) Symptoms are; not listening, not completing tasks, impulsiveness and easy distraction making school work difficult. People with ADHD are continuously moving, climbing and jumping. Their concentration is extremely limited. Medication is administered where it can be helpful. Keeping chemically free is important. Chemicals are additives such as artificial dyes, preservatives, extracts, sulfates, and hydrogenated oils. Avoid sugars and caffeine for obvious reasons. This is a good reason to cook at home, knowing what chemicals you put into your foods.

ILLNESS (Cont.)

<u>Hypoglycemia and Hyperglycemia</u> Thresholds for glucose are different than normal levels. Below normal level is hypoglycemia. Above normal is hyperglycemia. Symptoms are being light headed, headaches, fatigue, mood swings (depression, irritability) and a craving for starches. This all applies to both conditions. Diets have a direct effect on people with these conditions. High protein/low carbohydrate diets are sometimes recommended. Unlimited vegetables, meats (proteins) and fluids on a regular three hour schedule does wonders for the blood (sugar) levels and the spirit. Keep carbs low and controlled. It is better <u>not</u> to eat sugars, white flours, caffeine, alcohol and limit fruits. Keep in mind that Lima beans and corn are vegetables that are considered starches. Also grapes and pineapples are higher in sugar content.

<u>Candidas</u> Symptoms are very similar to hypoglycemia with headaches, mood swings, fatigue, irritability, bloating and craving for starches. People with this condition need to utilize vitamins to boost the immune system. Eliminate white sugars, white flours, fruits, molds and yeasts from the diet (see allergy list). Caffeine, alcohol and smoking are prohibited.

<u>Stomach Ulcers</u> People with ulcer disorders need to keep sailing smoothly. Bland diets are recommended with no spicy or fried foods. Soft foods like eggs, cooked cereals, soups, and pureed vegetables are recommended to settle disturbances.

<u>Pregnancy</u> With births increasing, the stomach needs a little attention too. Morning sickness during pregnancy does pose problems for eating nutritious foods (OR food at all). Strong smelling and spicy foods cause quite a bit of trouble here. All nutrients need to be increased for the duration of the pregnancy with extra proteins and vitamins (Check Vitamin and Mineral Chart). Easy and quick to prepare foods are suggested, along with drinking fluids <u>in between</u> meals and snacks.

<u>Celiac Disease</u> or Gluten Sensitive affects children up to the age of 6 years old and adults. Omitting all gluten (barley, oats, rye and wheat) in any form is recommended. A diet of rice, meats, vegetables, fruits, eggs and cheeses if tolerated is prescribed. The thickeners that can be used are cornstarch, Arrowroot or potato flour. Sugar is fine if tolerated. One needs to be aware of iron deficiency anemia so plan a diet high in iron (See Chart on Vitamins).

BUT I CAN'T EAT THAT

ILLNESS (Cont.)

IBS (Irritable Bowel Syndrome) and upper intestinal problems such as Crones Disease need to watch for iron deficiencies and anemia. Due to much fluid loss, a bland diet is recommended for therapy with foods rich in iron. Light soups, cooked soft foods and vegetables, boiled, broiled or baked meats, rice, noodles, potatoes, cooked or canned fruit are good. Refrain from drinking alcohol.

Cancer Unfortunately this devastating disease affects 1,040,000 people in the USA and the statistics are growing. This has the worst side effects of all diseases today. There are many different kinds of cancers. Some interfere with the absorption and digestion of proteins, minerals and fats in the body. Some treatments are just as extreme. Anorexia with no will to eat, iron anemia, potassium losses and B-12 deficiencies become a real threat. Recommended therapy is:

Bland diets to reduce any gastric stress

Nutritious non-acidic foods

Non irritating spices

Easy to prepare meals

Easy to swallow courses

Foods containing vitamins A, E, C, B-12

Multiple vitamin supplements

Electrolytes are beneficial

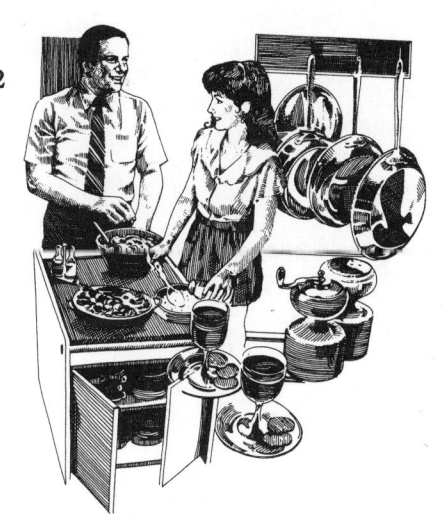

INDEX

APPLE — 111–114, 158
- Allergy Apple Pie — 161
- Apple Envelope — 166
- Baked Whole Fruit — 159
- BASIC: Apple Leather — 159
- Breakfast Apple Fritters — 171
- Breakfast Delight — 115
- Butter — 113
- Jello — 114
- German Apple Pancakes — 63
- Puff — 114
- Smoothie — 112
- Applesauce — 111
- Crock Pot Applesauce — 111
- Microwaved Applesauce — 111
- Muffins — 98
- Tips, Applesauce — 112

BEEF — 29–44
- All Homemade Lasagna — 35
- Allergy Lasagna — 36
- Beef Chow Mein — 23
- Beef, Quick Meal Ideas — 41
- Beef, Leftover Pie — 29
- Beef Seasoning — 142
- Beef Stew — 27
- BASIC: Beef Stock (Oxtail) — 133
- Extra Savory Meat Loaf — 24
- Flank Steak — 29
- Hamburger — 30
- Hamburger Bake — 32
- Hamburger Skillet Toss — 31
- Heidi's Allergy Pot Roast — 25
- Meat Stuffed Zucchini — 33
- One Meal Salad — 130
- Porcupine Balls — 24
- Pureed Meat — 34
- S.O.M. (More Save Our Mouth) — 28
- Swiss Steak — 26

BISCUITS — 90–91
- BBP — 91
- Cut — 90
- Drop — 90
- RBP — 91

INDEX

BREADS	82-86
Basic: French	83
Corn	82
Croutons	149
Cut Biscuits-w/ French Bread Basic	83
Drop	88
Green	84
Heavier English Muffin Bread	86
Italian	84
Orange	85
Red	84
Rye Allergy Loaf	89
Sticks	84
Zucchini	87
Zucchini-w/ Brown Rice Flour	86
BUTTERS	
Apple Butter	113
Clarified Butter	154
Herbal Butter	144
Peach Butter	115
Sesame Butter	144
CARROT	116-117
Baked Shredded Carrots	116
Carrot Dressing	149
Carrot Sauce	117
Grated Carrot Salad	116
Shredded Carrot Salad	129
Sweet Thins	117
CAULIFLOWER	
Basic: Cauliflower Soup	118
CELERY IDEAS	126
Boiled	126
Celery Soup	144
Cream of Celery Soup	144
Microwaved	126
Steamed	126
Stuffing	127
CHICKEN	46-60
Allergy Chow Mein	44
BASIC: Chicken Stock	132
Burgers	49
Breaded Strips	43
Chicken Seasoning	142

INDEX

CHICKEN (CONT.)
    Chicken Stock Ideas   138-140
        Basic: Cauliflower Soup   139
        Basic: Sweet Pea Soup   140
        Celery Soup   138
        Chive Sauce   145
        Cream of Celery Soup   138
        Cream of Chicken Soup   138
        Cream of Spinach Soup   138
        Imperial Green Soup   140
        Spinach Soup   138
        Zucchini Soup   139
    Crispy Chips   55
    CROCK POT   39
        Browned   39
        Poached   39
        Roasted   39
        Not Browned   39
    Fritters   45
    Hot Salad   49
    Liver Pate   51
    Loaf   46-47
    Marinated Breasts   40
    No Fuss Dinner   48
    One Meal Salad   130
    One Step, and Rice   49
    Plain Baked   37
    Plain Microwaved   37
    Plain Oven Fried   37
    Pot Pie   42
    Protein Spread   50
    Quick   41
    Rice Scrapple   44
    Rolls   48
    Rolled Bundles   45
    Tomato Casserole   51
CORN   119
    Pancakes   119
    Smashed   119
DOUGH
    Allergy Pie Pastry   160

INDEX

EGGS	60-64
Allergy Angel Food Cake	167
Butter Cookies	175
Butterflies	174
Desert Rollups	57
Dunkin Eggs	54
Eatable Short Bread	176
Egg Times	52
Ideal Egg Uses	52-53
German Apple Pancakes	55
German Pancakes	54
Jonathan's Allergy Rollups	57
One Meal Salad	130
Skillet Breakfast	55
FISH	65-67
Captain J.R.'s Seafood Specialty	114
Fish Broth	137
Fish and Spinach Wraps	60
Fish Seasoning	143
Fried "Rice A Tuna"	113
No Turn Basic Fish Formulas	58-59
Baked	58
Baked and Stuffed	58
Broiled	58
Pan Fried	59
Sauce	59
Steak	59
Steamed	58
One Meal Salad	130
Seafood Pilaf	60
Tuna Patties	60
FRUIT	
Allergy Strawberry Pie	163
Allergy Peach Pie	164
Allergy Pineapple Pudding	169
Basic Drinks: Pop	152
Frozen Watermelon	115
Fruit Ideas	115
Jam Formula	113
Fruit Shake	152
Lite Watermelon Freeze	169
Peach Butter	115
Peach Sauce	145

INDEX

FRUIT (Cont.)
    Pear Sauce   146
    Quicker Sauces   113
    Salad Dressing for Fruits   129
    Simple Fruit Sauce   113
    Ultra Smooth Fruit Sauce   170
INGREDIENTS AND SUBSTITUTIONS FOR: 24–27
    Antacid   25
    Baking Powder   25
    Bread Crumbs   25
    Butter   25
    Cake Flour   24
    Egg   25
    Fresh Celery   24
    Fresh Onion   24
    Karo Syrup   25
    Wheat Flour   24
    Milk   25
    Non-Citric Mayo Spread   27
    Sugar   25
    Vanilla   25
LAMB   68–73
    Allergy Lamb Loaf   66
    Chops   61
    BASIC: Lamb Stock   134
    Meatballs in White Sauce   67
    One Meal Salad   130
    Pot Pie   62
    Roast   61
    Stew   64
    Wrap   65
LISTS, TABLES, CHARTS
    Cooking Nuts   154
    Cooking Times Over Charcoal   155
    Freezer Storage Time Table
    Microwave Hints   153–154
    Peak Seasons for Fresh Foods
    QUICK Cooking Times (Pressure Cooker)   156
    Recipe Charts   9–15
    Steaming Veggies Timetable   128
    Vitamins and Minerals

INDEX

MISCELLANEOUS
- Banana Dream Shake — 154
- Basic: Anything Goes Soup — 152
- Basic Drinks: Pop — 137
- Broccoli Marinade — 152
- Carrot Dressing — 190
- Cornmeal Drops — 149
- Croutons — 151
- Dragon Cookies — 149
- Flour Tortillas — 150
- Fructose Reduced Syrup — 102
- Fruit Shake — 17
- Heidi's No Cheese Ravioli — 152
- Homemade Peanut Butter — 80
- Homemade Peanut Butter Spread — 78
- Meat Turnovers — 78
- Pastry Dough (Meat Turnovers) — 99
- Non-Citric Mayo Spread — 99
- Nuts, Cooking — 27
- Pastry Dough (Pot Pies) — 154
- Rye Allergy Loaf — 99
- Rye Tortillas — 89

MUFFINS — 98–100
- Apple — 92
- Peach — 93
- Rice — 94
- Rye — 92
- Sweet Pineapple — 93

PANCAKES — 94–97
- Auntie's — 96
- Corn — 119
- Corn Pone — 94
- Fresh Corn — 95
- Green — 97
- Orange — 96
- Rice — 96
- Zucchini — 95
- Zucchini (Regular) — 95

PASTA
    Basic Pasta   98
    Fried Noodles   98
    Ravioli   98
    Spinach, Beets, Carrots, Tomato   98
    Vegetable Noodles   98
PORK   68–73
    Allergy Sausage Patties   70
    Basic Pork Chops   74
        Baked   68
        Braised   68
        Grilled   74
    Chop Skillet Dinner   73
    City Chicken   72
    Just Ribs (Western Spare Ribs)   69
    One Meal Salad   130
    Pot Pie with Vegetables   71
    Roast   69
    Sweet Pork Cutlets   70
    Tenderloin   68

INDEX

POTATOES	120
Cakes	120
Chips	121
Croutons	121
Fries	122
Plain Baked Potatoes	121
Skillet Hash Browns	122
RICE	103-109
Apple Breakfast Delight	109
Basic Brown Rice	104
Basic White Rice	103
Brown Rice Cakes	106
Captain J.R.'s Seafood Specialty	108
Crock Pot Brown Rice	105
Fried "Rice A Tuna"	107
Herbs and Rice	106
Indian Wehani Rice	107-108
Ready Brown Rice	105
Sweet Peach Breakfast Rice	109
SALAD IDEAS	129
Carrot Dressing	149
One Meal Salad	130
Salad Dressing for Fruits	129
Shredded Carrot Salad	129
SAUCES	145-148
Allergy Spaghetti Sauce	148
Basic: Pan Drippings	141
Chive Sauce	48, 145
Gravies	141
Peach Sauce	145
Peanut Butter Sauce	145
Pear Sauce	146
Quicker Sauces	113
Simple Fruit Sauce	113
SEASONINGS	142-144
Beef Seasoning	142
Chicken Seasoning	142
Drying Herbs in Microwave	142
Fish Seasoning	143
Herbal Butter	144

INDEX

SEASONINGS (Cont.)
- Herbal Salt — 144
- Pizza Seasoning — 143
- Sesame Butter — 144
- Vegetable Seasoning — 143

SOUPS — 132–140
- BASIC: Anything Goes Soup — 137
- BASIC: Beef Stock (Oxtail) — 133
- BASIC: Chicken Stock — 132
- BASIC: Lamb Stock — 134
- BASIC: Vegetable Broth — 135
- Chunky Vegetable Soup — 135
- Cream of Broccoli Soup — 136
- Cream of Lettuce Soup — 135
- Fish Broth — 137
- Lite Lettuce Soup — 135
- Quick Broccoli Soup — 136
- Thicker Vegetable Soup — 135
- Vegetable Broth Ideas — 136
- CHICKEN STOCK IDEAS — 138
  - Basic: Cauliflower Soup — 139
  - Basic: Sweet Pea Soup — 140
  - Celery Soup — 138
  - Chive Sauce — 145
  - Cream of Celery Soup — 138
  - Cream of Chicken Soup — 138
  - Cream of Spinach Soup — 138
  - Imperial Green Soup — 140
  - Spinach Soup — 138
  - Zucchini Soup — 139

SUBSTITUTIONS — 16–19
- Antacid, natural — 19
- Baking Powder — 18
- Bread Crumbs — 18
- Butter — 18
- Cake Flour — 16
- Celery — 18
- Egg — 16
- Milk — 17
  - Oat Milk — 17
  - Using egg whites — 17
  - Zucchini Milk — 17

INDEX

SUBSTITUTIONS (Cont.)
- Non-Citric Mayo Spread — 19
- Onion — 18
- Sugar: Fructose Reduced Syrup — 17
- Vanilla — 18
- Water — 19
- Wheat Flour — 16

SWEET MEAL TOPPERS — 158-176
- Allergy Angel Food Cake — 167
- Allergy Apple Pie — 161
- Apples — 158
- Apple Envelope — 166
- Allergy Peach Pie — 164
- Allergy Pie Pastry — 160
- Allergy Pineapple Pudding — 169
- Allergy Pizzelles — 173
- Allergy Strawberry Pie — 163
- Baked Whole Fruit — 159
- BASIC: Apple Leather — 159
- Breakfast Apple Fritters — 171
- Butter Cookies — 175
- Butterflies — 174
- Crisp Rice Treats — 177
- Customized Granola — 168
- Dragon Cookies — 150
- Eatable Short Bread — 176
- Fructose Reduced Syrup — 168
- Lite Allergy Pumpkin Pie — 165
- Lite Watermelon Freeze — 169
- Ultra Smooth Fruit Sauce — 170

TURKEY — 76-77
- C/T Meatballs — 77
- Ground Turkey — 77
- Hash — 76

VEAL — 74-75
- Patties (Plain) — 74
- Patties (Spiced) — 74
- Scallopini Cacciatore — 75

VEGETABLES — 124
- Basic: Cauliflower Soup — 139
- Basic: Vegetable Broth — 135
- Chunky Vegetable Soup — 135
- Cream of Broccoli Soup — 136

INDEX

VEGETABLES (Cont.)	
Cream of Lettuce Soup	135
Creamy Spinach	125
Herbal Vegetable Sauté	127
Lite Lettuce Soup	135
Lite Allergy Pumpkin Pie	165
Quick Broccoli Soup	136
Stir Fry Bok Choy w/ Napa Cabbage	125
Thicker Vegetable Soup	135
Your Favorite Veggies with Curry	124
Vegetable Seasoning	143
Vegetable Recipes:	
See SOUP, BREAD, PASTA and Individual Vegetable	
Headings	
WAFFLES	101
Allergy	101
Blueberry OR Fruit	101
Carob	101
Carob Chip	101
Chocolate	101
ZUCCHINI	123
Bread	93
Bread w/Brown Rice Flour	92
Broiled	123
Cakes	123
Microwaved	123
Pancakes	102
Pancakes (Regular)	102

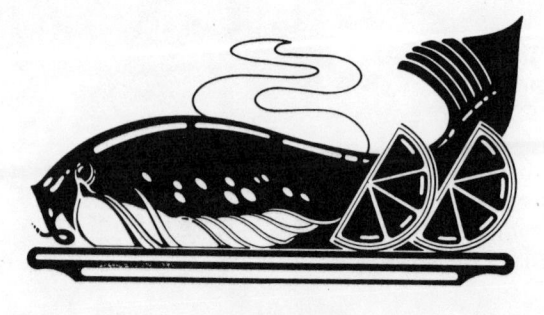

BUT I CAN'T EAT THAT

INDEX for Chapter 7-COMPANY'S COMING

Non-Allergy Recipes   181-198

APPETIZERS
- Vegetable Dip-Curry   178
- Dips   178
- KAY'S Cheese Ball   179
- Marianne's Chicken Drumetts   179
- Pepperoni Pizza Bread   180
- Split Pea Soup   181
- Vegetable Dip-Dill   178

BEEF, CHEESE, CHICKEN, EGG
- Cheese Broccoli Casserole   186
- Chicken, Royal   183
- Plain Good Beef Stew   182
- Sandra's Two Cheese Strata   185
- Sharon's Company Casserole   182
- Strata, Meat   185
- Strata, Vegetable   185
- Sweet and Sour Eggs   184

JELLO
- Family's Favorite Jello   191
- Lime Supreme (Jello)   191

VEGETABLES
- Broccoli Marinade   186
- Cheese Broccoli Casserole   186
- Strata, Vegetable   189

SWEETS
- Boston Cream Pie   191
- Carrot and Pineapple Cake   194
- Cream Cheese Cake   190
- Cream Cheese Frosting   198
- Family's Favorite Jello   187
- Fudge Melt Away's   193
- Great Pie Crust   188
- Lime Supreme (Jello)   187
- Mother-in-Law's Coffee Cake   189
- Potato Chip Cookies   192
- Walnut Bars   192

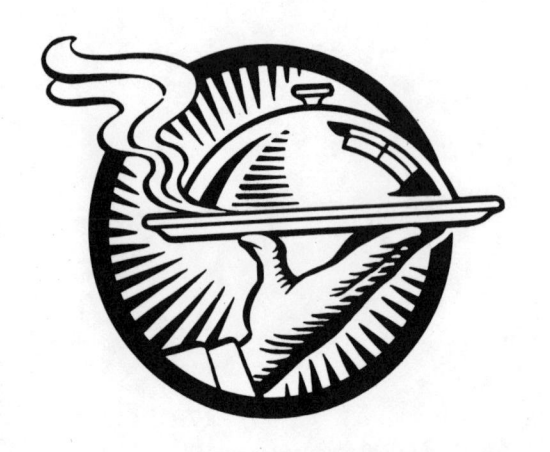

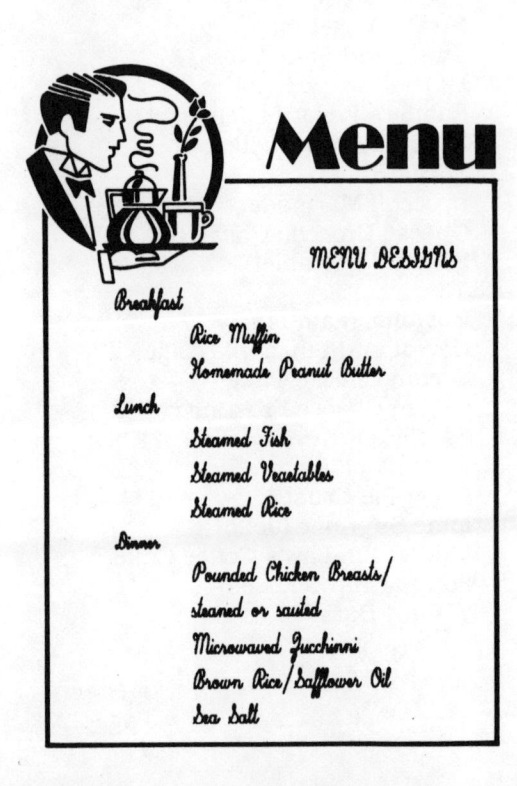

BUT I CAN'T EAT THAT

Menu

MENU DESIGNS

Breakfast
    Rice Muffin
    Homemade Peanut Butter

Lunch
    Steamed Fish
    Steamed Vegetables
    Steamed Rice

Dinner
    Pounded Chicken Breasts/
    steamed or sauted
    Microwaved Zucchinni
    Brown Rice/Safflower Oil
    Sea Salt

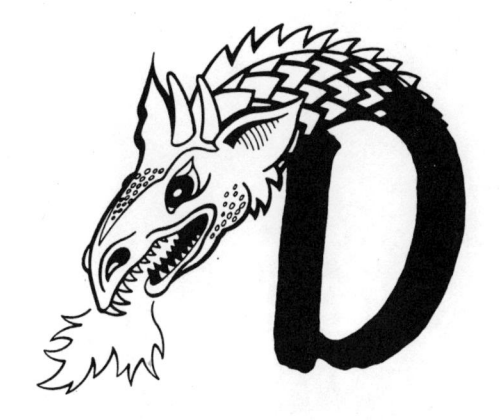

BUT I CAN'T EAT THAT

D

BUT I CAN'T EAT THAT

NOTES

BUT I CAN'T EAT THAT

NOTES

BUT I CAN'T EAT THAT

Dragon Express Press

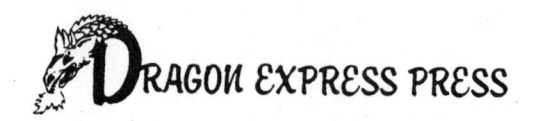

ORDER FORM

Fill in Order Form Below

Send To:
DRAGON EXPRESS PRESS
2604 Saybrook Road
University Hts., Ohio 44118-4722

Please mail me _____ copies of the Cookbook **But I Can't Eat That!** at $19.99 per copy. Add $4.00 for shipping/handling and $.50 per additional book ordered. Ohio residents please include 7% state tax. Enclosed is a check or money order for $_____.

```
No. of books ___ X $19.99 =        _____
Ohio State Tax 7%                  _____
              Sub Total            _____
Ship/Handling                      + 4.00
Shipping for Extra Books .50 ea.   _____
              TOTAL                _____
```

Mail my books to:
Name_____
Address_____
City, State, Zip_____

(Allow 4-6 weeks for delivery.)
Make checks payable to Dragon Express Press.

P.S.- Do you know someone this Cookbook will help? A book is a loving gift. Lift their spirits and give **But I Can't Eat That**! for Birthday or Holiday Gifts.

- Inquire about discount quantity book orders.